- Tast buds
- Pg 79 John
- sensation of the touch torque.

High-Yield Cell and Molecular Biology

High-Yield Cell and Molecular Biology

Ronald W. Dudek, Ph.D.
Department of Anatomy and Cell Biology
East Carolina University
School of Medicine
Greenville, North Carolina

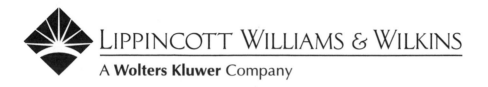

LIPPINCOTT WILLIAMS & WILKINS
A **Wolters Kluwer** Company

Editor: Elizabeth A. Nieginski
Editorial Director, Textbooks: Julie P. Scardiglia
Managing Editor: Darrin Kiessling
Marketing Manager: Jennifer Conrad
Development Editors: Karla M. Schroeder and Rosanne Hallowell
Illustrator: Kimberly A. Battista

351 West Camden Street
Baltimore, Maryland 21201-2436 USA

227 East Washington Square
Philadelphia, PA 19106

Printed in the United States of America

Library of Congress Cataloging-in-Publication Data

Dudek, Ronald W., 1950–
    High-yield cell and molecular biology / Ronald W. Dudek.
      p.   cm.—(High-yield series)
    ISBN 0-683-30359-7
    1. Molecular biology Outlines, syllabi, etc.   2. Pathology
Outlines, syllabi, etc.   3. Cytology Outlines, syllabi, etc.
    I. Title.   II. Series.
    QH506.D83   1999
    572.8—dc21   99-23316
                                   CIP

To purchase additional copies of this book, call our customer service department at **(800) 638-3030** or fax orders to **(301) 824-7390.** International customers should call **(301) 714-2324.**

  99 00 01 02 03
  1 2 3 4 5 6 7 8 9 10

Dedication

This book is affectionately dedicated to my good friend Ron Cicinelli. In our 30 years of friendship I have witnessed his dedication to family and friends. Ron brings a unique combination of strength and kindness to every personal interaction. I am honored to know him and wish that all of you could know him too. His life has been, and continues to be, a "high-yield" life.

Contents

Preface

The impact of molecular biology today and in the future cannot be underestimated. Gene therapy and cloning of sheep are explained and discussed in the daily newspapers. The clinical and etiological aspects of diseases are now being explained at the molecular biology level. Drugs that will have an impact on molecular biological processes are being designed right now by pharmaceutical companies for the treatment of various diseases and conditions (e.g., cancer, obesity). Molecular biology will be increasingly represented on the USMLE Step 1 exam.

How will medical schools teach the clinical relevance of molecular biology to our future physicians? Medical school curricula are already filled with needed and relevant "traditional" courses. Where will the time needed to teach a molecular biology course be found? I suspect what will happen is that many of the "traditional" courses will extend their discussion of various topics down to the molecular biology level. This approach will work, but it will in effect make molecular biology somewhat disjointed. The student will learn some molecular biology in a biochemistry course, some in a microbiology course, some in a histology course, and so forth. The problem this presents for the student reviewing for USMLE Step 1 is that the molecular biology information will be scattered among various course notes.

The solution: *High-Yield Cell and Molecular Biology*. Under one cover I have consolidated the important clinical issues related to molecular biology that are obvious "grist-for-the-mill" for USMLE Step 1 questions. It is my feeling that *High-Yield Cell and Molecular Biology* will be of tremendous benefit to any student seriously reviewing for the USMLE Step 1.

Please send your feedback comments to me at dudek@brody.med.ecu.edu.

Ronald W. Dudek, PhD

1

Packaging of Chromosomal DNA

I. NUCLEIC ACIDS [deoxyribonucleic acid (DNA) and ribonucleic acid (RNA)] consist of nucleotides which are composed of **(Figure 1-1):**

A. Nitrogenous bases

   1. Purines
      a. Adenine (A)
      b. Guanine (G)

   2. Pyrimidines
      a. Cytosine (C)
      b. Thymine (T)
      c. Uracil (U), which is found in RNA

B. Sugars

   1. Deoxyribose

   2. Ribose, which is found in RNA

C. Phosphate

II. THE HUMAN GENOME is all of the genetic information stored in the chromosomes of a human. It contains approximately 3×10^9 nucleotide pairs organized as 23 chromosomes.

III. CHROMOSOMES contain:

A. Specialized nucleotide sequences

   1. The **centromere** is a nucleotide sequence that binds to the mitotic spindle during cell division.

   2. The **telomere** is a nucleotide sequence located at the end of a chromosome. It allows replication of the full length of linear DNA (i.e., the DNA does not shorten with each replication cycle).

   3. **Replication origins** are nucleotide sequences that act as origination sites for replication. A human chromosome contains **numerous replication origins.**

B. **Bands.** Bands contain genes and are identified with fluorescent dyes and Giemsa stain.

   1. G bands are rich in A–T nucleotide pairs; they stain dark.

   2. R bands are rich in G–C nucleotide pairs; they stain light.

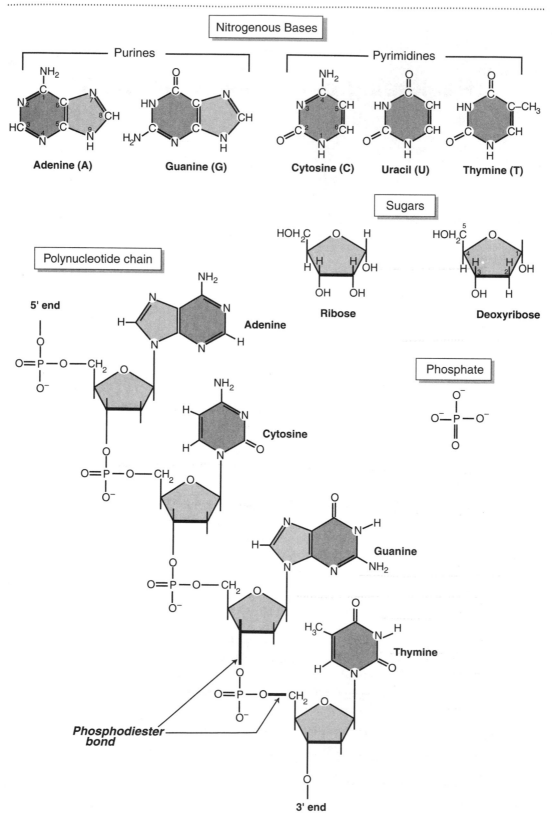

Nitrogenous Bases

Purines

Adenine (A)   Guanine (G)

Pyrimidines

Cytosine (C)   Uracil (U)   Thymine (T)

Sugars

Ribose   Deoxyribose

Polynucleotide chain

Phosphate

5' end

Adenine

Cytosine

Guanine

Thymine

Phosphodiester bond

3' end

IV. GENES. A **gene** is a region of DNA that produces a functional RNA molecule.

    A. Gene size varies. For example:

      1. The insulin gene has 1.7×10^3 (approximately 1700) nucleotides.

      2. The low-density lipoprotein (LDL) receptor gene has 45×10^3 (approximately 45,000) nucleotides.

      3. The dystrophin gene has 2000×10^3 (approximately 200,000,000) nucleotides.

    B. Gene regions

      1. Noncoding regions (**introns;** "**intervening sequences**") make up a majority of the nucleotide sequences of a gene.

      2. Coding regions (**exons;** "**expression sequences**") make up a minority of the nucleotide sequences of a gene.

V. CHROMATIN (**Figure 1-2**) is a complex of histone and nonhistone proteins that is bound to DNA.

    A. H2A, H2B, H3, and H4 histone proteins

      1. Histone proteins are small and contain a high proportion of **lysine** and **arginine** amino acids. Lysine and arginine give the proteins a positive charge that enhances binding to negatively charged DNA.

      2. Histone proteins bind to DNA regions that are rich in A-T nucleotide pairs.

      3. Histone proteins bind to DNA as two full turns of DNA wind around a **histone octamer** (two each of H2A, H2B, H3, and H4 histone proteins) forming a **nucleosome** (the fundamental unit of chromatin packing).

    B. H1 histone protein joins nucleosomes to form a 30-nm fiber.

    C. Types of chromatin. Heterochromatin and **euchromatin** (**active** and **inactive**) are packed in the cell nucleus.

      1. Ten percent of the chromatin is highly condensed, **transcriptionally inactive heterochromatin.**

      2. Ninety percent of the chromatin is less condensed: ten percent is **transcriptionally active euchromatin** and eighty percent is **transcriptionally inactive euchromatin.**

    D. Degree of compaction

      1. Human chromosome 1 contains approximately 260,000,000 base pairs.

      2. The distance between each base pair is 0.34 nm.

      3. The DNA in chromosome 1 is 88,000,000 nm, or 88,000 μm long ($260{,}000{,}000 \times 0.34$ nm = 88,400,000 nm).

      4. During metaphase, the chromosomes condense, and the 88,000 μm of DNA is reduced to 10 μm, an 8800-fold compaction (**Figure 1-3**).

Figure 1-1.   Chemical structure of the components of DNA (purines, pyrimidines, sugars, and phosphate), which form a polynucleotide chain. Note the phosphodiester bond. (Adapted and redrawn from Marks DB: *Board Review Series: Biochemistry*, 3rd ed. Baltimore, Williams & Wilkins, 1998, pp. 46, 48. Used by permission of Lippincott Williams & Wilkins, Philadelphia, PA.)

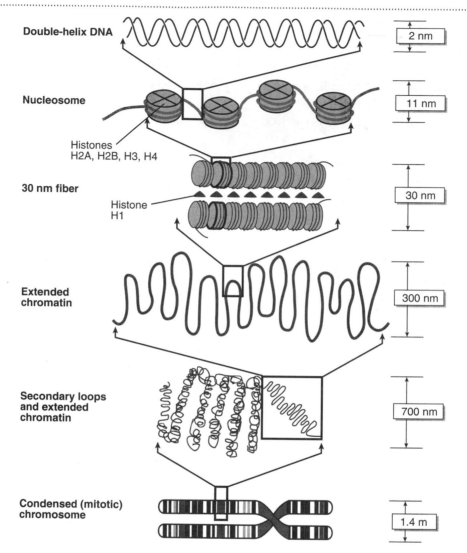

Figure 1-2. Levels of packaging of double-helix deoxyribonucleic acid (DNA) within a chromosome during metaphase. Double-helix DNA winds around a histone octamer of H2A, H2B, H3, and H4 histone proteins to form a nucleosome. Histone H1 joins the nucleosomes to form a 30 nm diameter fiber that consists of either extended chromatin or secondary loops within a condensed (mitotic) chromosome. (Adapted and redrawn with permission from Alberts B, Bray D, Johnson A et al: *Essential Cell Biology: An Introduction to the Molecular Biology of the Cell*. New York, Garland Publishing, 1998, p 354.)

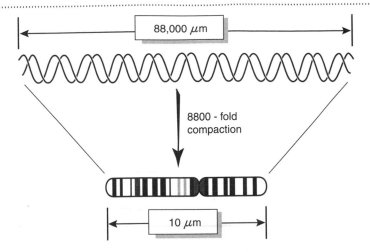

Figure 1-3.   Compaction of DNA in chromosome 1. When the double-helix DNA of chromosome 1 is unraveled, it is 88,000 μm long. When chromosome 1 condenses (as occurs during mitosis), the DNA is only 10 μm long (an 8800-fold compaction).

2

Chromosome Replication and DNA Synthesis

I. INTRODUCTION (Figure 2-1)

A. Chromosome replication occurs during the **S-phase** of the cell cycle. In S-phase, deoxyribonucleic acid (DNA) and histones are synthesized to form chromatin.

B. The structure of chromatin affects the timing of replication.

    1. DNA packaged as **heterochromatin** is replicated **late** in the S-phase. For example, in a female mammalian cell, the inactive X chromosome (Barr body) is packaged as **heterochromatin** and is replicated **late** in the S-phase. The active X chromosome is packaged as **euchromatin** and is replicated **early** in the S-phase.

    2. An **active gene** packaged as euchromatin is replicated **early** in the S-phase. For example, in the pancreatic beta cell, the insulin gene is replicated early in the S-phase. However, in other cell types (e.g., hepatocytes) in which the insulin gene is an **inactive gene,** the insulin gene is replicated **late in the S-phase.**

C. DNA polymerases require a **ribonucleic acid (RNA) primer** to begin DNA synthesis.

D. DNA polymerases copy a DNA template in the **3′ → 5′ direction.** New DNA strands are produced in the **5′ → 3′ direction.**

E. Deoxyribonucleoside 5′-triphosphates (dATP, dTTP, dGTP, dCTP) pair with the corresponding bases (i.e., A–T, G–C; see Chapter 1) on the template strand. They form a **phosphodiester bond with the 3′-OH group on the deoxyribose sugar,** which releases a **pyrophosphate.**

F. Replication is **semiconservative** (i.e., a molecule of double-helix DNA contains one intact parental DNA strand and one newly synthesized DNA strand).

II. A REPLICATION FORK (Figure 2-2) is a site at which DNA synthesis occurs.

A. Chromosome replication begins at specific nucleotide sequences **(replication origins)** that are located throughout the chromosome. Human DNA has **multiple replication origins** to ensure rapid DNA synthesis.

B. **DNA helicase** recognizes the replication origin. It opens the double helix at that site to form a **replication bubble** with a **replication fork** at each end.

C. A replication fork contains:

    1. A **leading strand** that is synthesized continuously by **DNA polymerase δ (delta).**

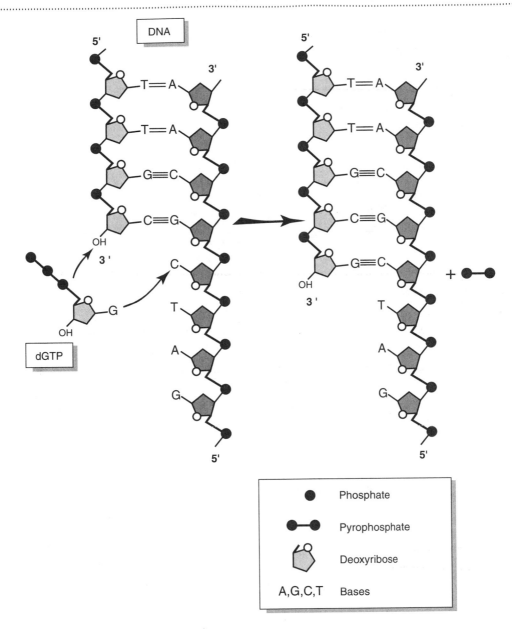

Figure 2-1. Addition of a deoxyribonucleoside 5′-triphosphate (*dGTP*) to the 3′-OH group of the growing deoxyribonucleic acid (*DNA*) strand and base pairing with cytosine during DNA synthesis. Note the release of pyrophosphate. (Adapted and redrawn from Marks DB: *Board Review Series: Biochemistry,* 3rd ed. Baltimore, Williams & Wilkins, 1998, p 56. Used by permission of Lippincott Williams & Wilkins, Philadelphia, PA.)

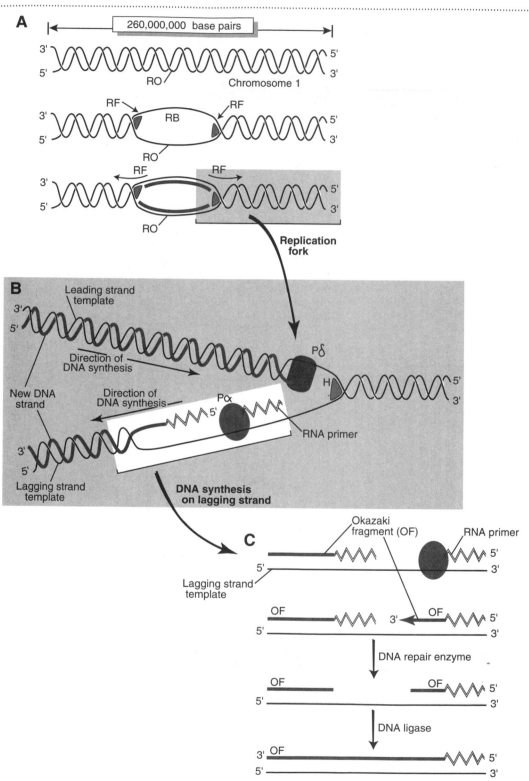

A

260,000,000 base pairs

3'
5'
RO
Chromosome 1

3'
5'
RF   RB   RF
RO

3'
5'
RF   RF
RO

Replication fork

B

Leading strand template
3'
5'
Direction of DNA synthesis
Pδ
H
5'
3'

New DNA strand
Direction of DNA synthesis
Pα
5'
RNA primer
3'
5'
Lagging strand template

DNA synthesis on lagging strand

C

Okazaki fragment (OF)   RNA primer
5'
3'
Lagging strand template

OF   OF
5'   3'   5'
3'

DNA repair enzyme

OF   OF
5'   5'
3'

DNA ligase

3' OF
5'   5'
3'

    2. A lagging strand that is synthesized discontinuously by **DNA polymerase α (alpha).**
        a. DNA primase synthesizes short RNA primers along the lagging strand.
        b. DNA polymerase α uses the RNA primer to synthesize DNA fragments called **Okazaki fragments.**
        c. Okazaki fragments end when they meet a downstream RNA primer.
        d. To form a continuous DNA strand from the Okazaki fragments, a **DNA repair enzyme** replaces the RNA primers with DNA.
        e. DNA ligase joins the DNA fragments.

D. If human chromosome 1 had only one replication origin, the rate of cell division would be severely decreased.

    1. Assume that human chromosome 1 contains 260,000,000 base pairs, the replication origin is located at the exact **center** of the chromosome, and DNA synthesis occurs at a rate of 100 base pairs/second.

    2. Two replication forks form (one at each end of the replication bubble). Each replication fork replicates 130,000,000 base pairs because the replication origin is located at the center of chromosome 1.

    3. The total time needed to replicate chromosome 1 is 1,300,000 seconds, or approximately **15 days** (130,000,000 base pairs ÷ 100 base pairs/second = 1,300,000 seconds). The S-phase of the human cell cycle is normally **8 hours,** which means that human DNA has multiple replication origins.

III. A TELOMERE is a nucleotide sequence **(in humans, GGGTTA)** at the end of a chromosome. The telomere allows replication of linear DNA to its full length.

A. DNA polymerases cannot synthesize in the 3′ → 5′ direction or initiate synthesis de novo. Therefore, removing the RNA primers leaves the 5′ end of the lagging strand shorter than the leading strand.

B. If the 5′ end of the lagging strand is not lengthened, the chromosome shortens each time the cell divides. This shortening causes cell death and may be related to the aging process in humans.

C. The enzyme **telomerase** recognizes the GGGTTA sequence on the leading strand and adds repeats of the sequence to the leading strand.

D. After the repeats are added to the leading strand, **DNA polymerase** α uses them as a template to synthesize the complementary repeats on the lagging strand. Thus, the lagging strand is lengthened.

Figure 2-2.   Replication fork. (A) Double-helix deoxyribonucleic acid (DNA) [*chromosome 1*] at a replication origin (*RO*) site. DNA helicase (*H*) binds at the RO and unwinds the double helix into two DNA strands. This site is called a replication bubble (*RB*). A replication fork (*RF*) forms at each end. DNA synthesis occurs bidirectionally from each replication fork (*arrows*). (B) Enlarged view of a replication fork. The leading strand is a template for continuous DNA synthesis in the 5′ → 3′ direction with DNA polymerase δ (*Pδ*). The lagging strand acts as a template for discontinuous DNA synthesis in the 5′ → 3′ direction with DNA polymerase α (*Pα*). DNA synthesis on the leading and lagging strands occurs in the 5′ → 3′ direction, but physically occurs in the opposite direction. (C) DNA synthesis on the lagging strand proceeds differently than on the leading strand. DNA primase synthesizes RNA primers. DNA polymerase α uses these ribonucleic acid (*RNA*) primers to synthesize DNA, or Okazaki, fragments (*OF*). Okazaki fragments end when they join a downstream RNA primer. DNA repair enzymes replace the RNA primers with DNA. Finally, DNA ligase joins the Okazaki fragments.

E. <u>DNA ligase</u> joins the repeats to the lagging strand. A **nuclease** cleaves the ends to form double-helix DNA with flush ends.

IV. DAMAGE AND REPAIR OF DNA. DNA repair involves <u>DNA excision</u> of the damaged site, <u>DNA synthesis</u> of the correct sequence, and **DNA ligation.**

A. Depurination

    1. Each day, the DNA of each human cell loses approximately 5000 purines (A or G) when the N-glycosyl bond between the purine and the deoxyribose sugar phosphate is broken.

    2. Depurination is the most common type of damage to DNA. When it occurs, the deoxyribose sugar phosphate is missing a purine base.

    3. To begin repair, **AP (apurinic site) endonuclease** recognizes the site of the missing purine and nicks the deoxyribose sugar phosphate.

    4. A **phosphodiesterase** excises the deoxyribose sugar phosphate.

    5. **DNA polymerase** and **DNA ligase** restore the correct DNA sequence and heal the nick in the strand.

B. Deamination of cytosine (C) to uracil (U) ✓

    1. Each day, approximately 100 cytosines spontaneously deaminate to uracil.

    2. If the uracil is not restored to cytosine, then at replication, an incorrect U–A base pairing occurs instead of a correct C–G base pairing.

    3. To begin repair, the enzyme **uracil–DNA glycosidase** recognizes and removes uracil. It does not remove thymine because thymine is distinguished from uracil by a **methyl group on carbon 5.**

    4. An **AP (apyriminic site) endonuclease** recognizes the site of the missing base and nicks the deoxyribose sugar phosphate.

    5. A **phosphodiesterase** excises the deoxyribose sugar phosphate.

    6. **DNA polymerase** and **DNA ligase** restore the correct DNA sequence and heal the nick in the strand.

C. Pyrimidine dimerization

    1. Sunlight [ultraviolet (UV) radiation] causes covalent linkage of adjacent pyrimidines, forming, for example, **thymine dimers.**

    2. To begin repair, the **uvrABC enzyme** recognizes the pyrimidine dimer and excises a 12-residue oligonucleotide that includes the dimer.

    3. **DNA polymerase** and **DNA ligase** restore the correct DNA sequence and heal the nick in the strand.

V. THE CLINICAL IMPORTANCE OF DNA REPAIR MECHANISMS is illustrated by the following rare inherited diseases that involve genetic defects in DNA repair enzymes:

A. Xeroderma pigmentosum (XP)

    1. XP causes hypersensitivity to **sunlight (UV radiation)** and, as a result, severe skin lesions and skin cancer. Most patients die before they are 30 years old.

2. XP is probably caused by an inability to remove pyrimidine dimers, most likely because of a genetic defect in one or more enzymes involved in their removal. In humans, removal of these dimers requires at least eight gene products.

B. Ataxia-telangiectasia

  1. Ataxia-telangiectasia causes hypersensitivity to **ionizing radiation** and, as a result, cerebellar ataxia, oculocutaneous telangiectasia, and immunodeficiency.

  2. Ataxia-telangiectasia is probably caused by defects in the enzymes involved in DNA repair.

C. Fanconi's anemia

  1. Fanconi's anemia causes hypersensitivity to **DNA cross-linking agents** and, as a result, leukemia and progressive aplastic anemia.

  2. Fanconi's anemia is probably caused by defects in the enzymes involved in DNA repair.

D. Bloom syndrome

  1. Bloom syndrome causes hypersensitivity to **many DNA-damaging agents** and, as a result, immunodeficiency, growth retardation, and predisposition to cancer.

  2. Bloom syndrome is probably caused by widespread defects in the enzymes involved in DNA repair.

E. Hereditary nonpolyposis colorectal cancer (HNPCC)

  1. Although most colorectal cancers are not caused by genetic factors, HNPCC accounts for 15% of all cases of colorectal cancer.

  2. The HNPCC gene (the human homologue to the *Escherichia coli* **mutS** and **mutL** genes that code for DNA repair enzymes) is involved in HNPCC.

  3. Identification of the genes responsible for HNPCC permits early detection by genetic testing. Early diagnosis improves survival because the early stage of HNPCC is the outgrowth of small benign polyps that are easily removed.

3
Genetic Recombination

I. INTRODUCTION. Although DNA replication and repair is crucial to cell survival, it does not explain human genetic variability. Some of the variability is imported by DNA rearrangements that are caused by **genetic recombination,** either general or site-specific.

II. GENERAL RECOMBINATION (Figure 3-1A) involves **single-stranded DNA** and requires **DNA sequence homology.**

- **A.** An important example of general recombination occurs during **"crossing over,"** when two homologous chromosomes pair during **meiosis** (gamete formation).
- **B.** RecBCD protein makes single-strand nicks in DNA to form single-stranded "whiskers."
- **C. Single-strand binding (SSB)** protein stabilizes the single-stranded DNA.
- **D.** During **synapsis, RecA** protein allows the single strand to invade and interact with the double- helix DNA of the other chromosome. This interaction requires DNA sequence homology.
- **E.** A DNA strand on the homologous chromosome repeats this process to form an important intermediate structure (**crossover exchange,** or **Holliday junction**) that has two crossing strands and two noncrossing strands.
- **F.** The two crossing strands are cut, and DNA repair produces two homologous chromosomes with exchanged DNA segments.

III. SITE-SPECIFIC RECOMBINATION (Figure 3-1B) involves the insertion of **double-stranded DNA.**

- **A.** An important example of site-specific recombination is the insertion of **viral DNA** into host DNA.
- **B.** Many DNA viruses and other transposable elements (see Chapter 4) encode for a recombination enzyme called **integrase** or **transposase,** respectively.
- **C.** Integrase recognizes specific nucleotide sequences and cuts the viral DNA.
- **D.** The cut ends of the viral DNA attack and break the host double-helix DNA.
- **E.** The viral DNA is inserted into the host DNA.
- **F.** DNA repair occurs to fill the gaps.

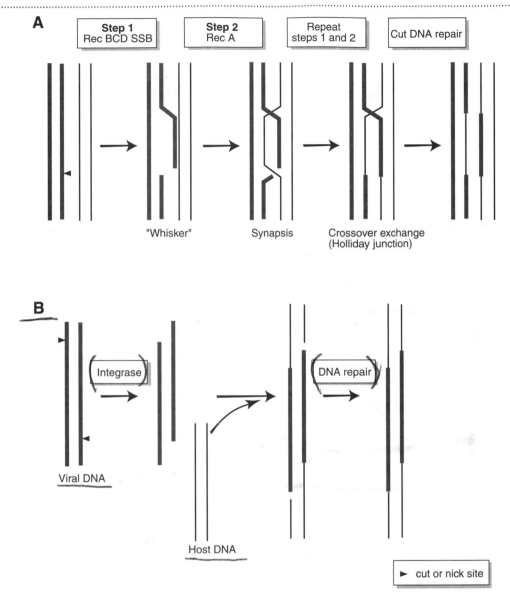

Figure 3-1.   The two types of genetic recombination. (A) General recombination during meiosis. (B) Site-specific recombination during deoxyribonucleic acid (DNA) viral infection. RecBCD = a protein discovered in E. coli that is essential for general **rec**ombination; SSB = single-strand binding; RecA = a protein discovered in E. coli that is encoded by the recA (**rec**ombination) gene.

4

Transposable Elements

I. INTRODUCTION

A. Transposable elements are <u>mobile deoxyribonucleic acid (DNA) sequences</u> that jump from one place in the genome to another **(transposition).** The cause of transposition is unclear.

B. Nine percent of the human genome consists of two families of transposable elements:

1. <u>Alu sequences</u> account for 5% of the human genome and are 300 base pairs long.

2. <u>LINE-1 sequences</u> account for 4% of the human genome and are 6000 base pairs long.

C. Transposable elements undergo long quiescent periods followed by periods of intense movement **(transposition bursts).** These bursts contribute to the genetic variability of the genome.

II. MECHANISMS OF TRANSPOSITION. Transposable elements jump either directly as double-stranded DNA or through a ribonucleic acid (RNA) intermediate.

A. Double-stranded DNA (Figure 4-1A)

1. Transposase is a recombination enzyme similar to integrase. It cuts the transposable element at sites marked by **inverted repeat DNA sequences** that are approximately 20 base pairs long. Transposase is encoded in the DNA of the transposable element.

2. The transposable element is inserted at a new location, possibly on another chromosome.

3. This mechanism is similar to the one that a **DNA virus** uses to transform host DNA (see Chapter 3).

B. <u>RNA intermediate (see Figure 4-1B)</u>

1. The transposable element undergoes transcription, which produces an RNA copy that encodes a reverse transcriptase enzyme.

2. **Reverse transcriptase** uses the RNA copy to produce a double-stranded DNA copy of the transposable element.

3. The transposable element is inserted at a new location by a mechanism similar to the one that an **RNA virus (retrovirus)** uses to transform host DNA.

Figure 4-1. Mechanisms of transposition. (A) Transposition as double-stranded deoxyribonucleic acid *(DNA)*. (B) Transposition through a ribonucleic acid *(RNA)* intermediate. *TE* = transposable element; *RT* = RNA code for reverse transcriptase.

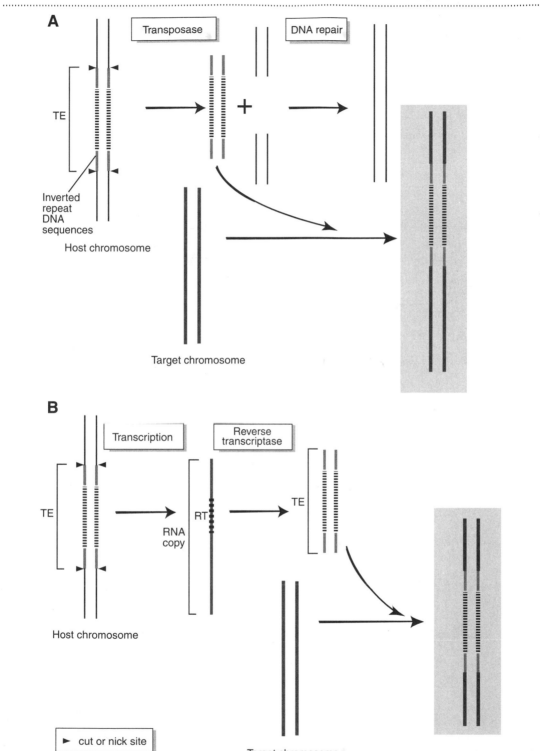

A

Transposase

DNA repair

TE

Inverted
repeat
DNA
sequences

Host chromosome

Target chromosome

B

Transcription

Reverse
transcriptase

TE

RNA
copy

RT

TE

Host chromosome

► cut or nick site

Target chromosome

III. TRANSPOSABLE ELEMENTS AND GENETIC VARIABILITY (Figure 4-2). Transposable elements affect the genetic variability of an organism in several ways:

A. Mutation at the former site of the transposable element (see Figure 4-2A)

    1. After transposase removes the transposable element from its site on the host chromosome, the host DNA undergoes DNA repair.

    2. A mutation may occur at the repair site.

B. Level of gene expression (see Figure 4-2B)

    1. If the transposable element moves to the target DNA near an active gene, the transposable element may affect the level of gene expression.

    2. Most of these changes in the level of gene expression would be detrimental to the organism. However, over time, some changes might be beneficial and spread through the population.

C. Gene inactivation (see Figure 4-2C). If the transposable element moves to the target DNA in the center of a gene sequence, the gene is mutated and inactivated.

D. Gene transfer (see Figure 4-2D)

    1. If two transposable elements are close together, the transposition mechanism may cut the ends of both of them.

    2. The DNA between the two transposable elements will move to a new location.

    3. If the DNA contains a gene, the gene is transferred to a new location.

    4. Gene transfer is especially important in the development of antibiotic resistance in bacteria. Transposable elements in bacterial DNA can move to bacteriophage DNA, which can spread to other bacteria. For example, if the bacterial DNA between the two transposable elements contains the gene for tetracycline resistance, then the recipient bacterium becomes resistant to tetracycline.

Figure 4-2.   Effect of transposable elements on genetic variability. (A) Mutation at the former site of the transposable element (TE). (B) Effect on the level of gene expression. (C) Gene inactivation. (D) Gene transfer. DNA = deoxyribonucleic acid; Tet^R = gene for tetracycline resistance.

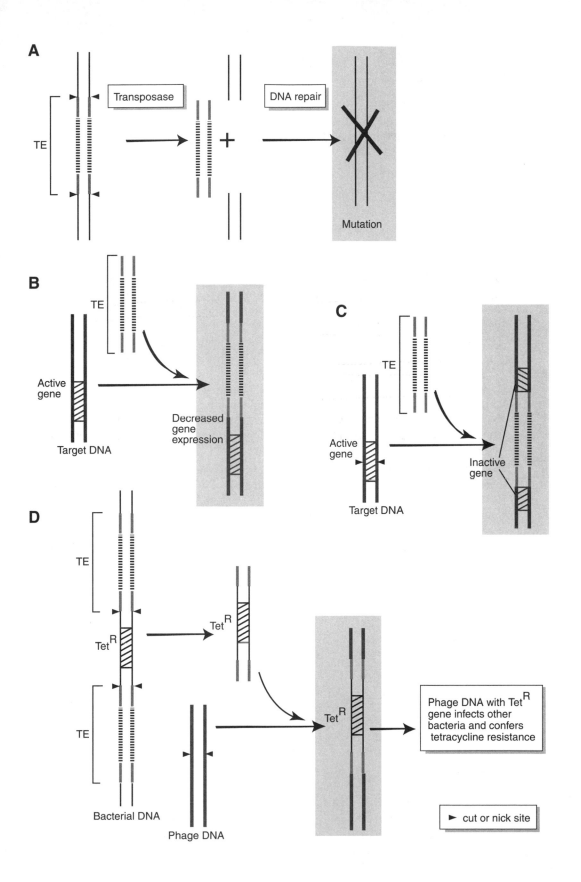

A

Transposase

DNA repair

TE

Mutation

B

TE

Active gene

Target DNA

Decreased gene expression

C

TE

Active gene

Target DNA

Inactive gene

D

TE

Tet^R

TE

Tet^R

Bacterial DNA

Phage DNA

Tet^R

Phage DNA with Tet^R gene infects other bacteria and confers tetracycline resistance

▶ cut or nick site

5

Gene Amplification

I. INTRODUCTION (Figure 5-1). Gene amplification occurs when repeated rounds of deoxyribonucleic acid (DNA) synthesis yield **multiple copies of a gene.** The copies are arranged as tandem arrays within a chromosome. Gene amplification usually results in increased levels of the protein that the gene encodes.

II. CLINICAL CONSIDERATIONS

    A. Drug resistance in cancer cells. Cancer cells may become resistant to **methotrexate,** a common chemotherapeutic agent. Methotrexate inhibits **dihydrofolate reductase,** which is involved in DNA synthesis. Cancer cells often become resistant to methotrexate through amplification of the dihydrofolate reductase gene. This amplification increases dihydrofolate reductase levels, which overcome effective inhibition by methotrexate.

    B. Amplification of genes involved in the cell cycle (proto-oncogenes). Proto-oncogene amplification contributes to uncontrolled cell growth and tumor development. (See Chapter 14.)

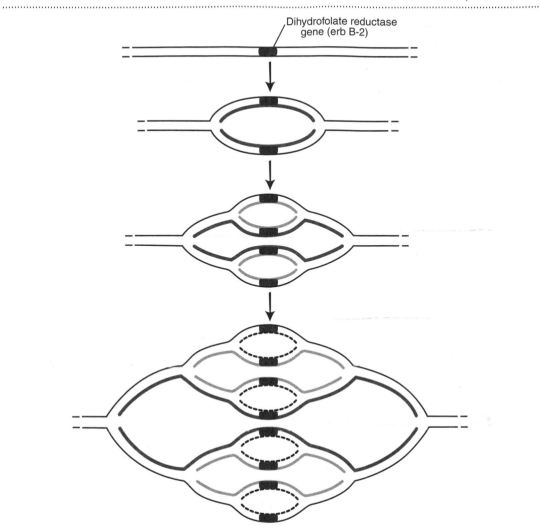

Figure 5-1.   Gene amplification.

6

Recombinant DNA Technology

I. INTRODUCTION. Laboratory procedures to **manipulate deoxyribonucleic acid (DNA)** [**recombinant DNA technology**] drove many important discoveries that affect clinical medicine. Understanding these discoveries requires an understanding of DNA laboratory procedures.

II. RESTRICTION ENZYMES (**Figure 6-1**) are bacterial enzymes that catalyze the **hydrolysis of the phosphodiester bond** in the DNA molecule (**cut the DNA**) at **specific nucleotide sequences** (4–10 base pairs). These enzymes are crucial to DNA technology because treating a specific DNA sample with a particular restriction enzyme always produces the same pattern of DNA fragments.

III. GEL ELECTROPHORESIS (**Figure 6-2**). After a DNA sample is fragmented with a restriction enzyme, the fragments are separated **by size** with gel electrophoresis. The sizes of the DNA fragments are compared, and a physical (**restriction**) map of the sample is constructed to show each cut site.

IV. ENZYMATIC METHOD OF DNA SEQUENCING (**Figure 6-3**). Restriction maps provide useful information about a DNA sample, but the ultimate physical map of DNA is its **nucleotide sequence,** which is established with **DNA sequencing.** This method combines DNA synthesis with **dideoxyribonucleoside triphosphates** that **lack the 3´-OH group** that they normally contain. If a dideoxyribonucleoside triphosphate is incorporated into DNA during DNA synthesis, addition of the next nucleotide is **blocked** because the 3´-OH group is missing. This blocking is the basis for the enzymatic method of DNA sequencing.

V. SOUTHERN BLOTTING AND PRENATAL TESTING FOR SICKLE CELL ANEMIA (**Figure 6-4**). Southern blotting uses a **DNA probe** and the **hybridization reaction** to identify a specific DNA sequence (e.g., the gene for the β-globin hemoglobin chain).

A. A **DNA probe** is a single-stranded DNA segment (an **oligonucleotide** with 10–120 base pairs) that participates in a hybridization reaction.

B. In a **hybridization reaction,** a single-stranded DNA segment (e.g., DNA probe) binds to or hybridizes with another single-stranded DNA segment that has a complementary nucleotide sequence. This reaction exploits a fundamental property of DNA to **denature** and **renature.** The double-helix DNA strands are joined by **weak hydrogen bonds** that are broken (denatured) by **high temperature** (90° C) or **alkaline pH** to

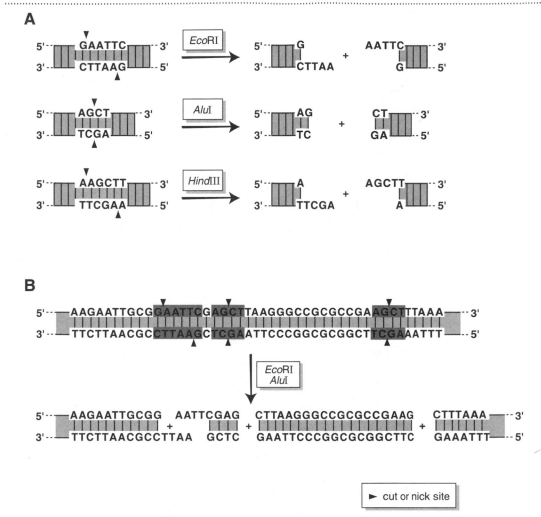

Figure 6-1. Action of restriction enzymes. (A) Hydrolysis of the phosphodiester bond by restriction enzymes *Eco*RI, *Alu*I, and *Hind*III. The specific nucleotide sequences recognized by each restriction enzyme and the cut sites (▲ ▼) are shown. *Eco*RI and *Hind*III produce DNA fragments that have staggered ends ("sticky"). *Alu*I produces DNA fragments that have blunt ends. (B) A long DNA sequence has many cut sites. If the same sequence is treated with both *Eco*RI and *Alu*I, the same four DNA fragments are always produced because the restriction enzymes are specific.

form single-stranded DNA. At **low temperature** or **acid pH,** double-helix DNA is reformed (renatured) from the single-stranded DNA.

C. Prenatal testing for sickle cell anemia (see Figure 6-4B). Gene cloning and sequencing permits the creation of a DNA probe that hybridizes with the gene (e.g., prenatal testing for sickle cell anemia). Sickle cell anemia is a recessive genetic disease that is caused by a mutation in the β-globin gene. This mutation converts a single amino acid in the β-globin protein from **glutamic acid** (normal) to **valine** (mutant). Because both the normal gene and the mutant gene have been sequenced, DNA probes can locate both genes with Southern blotting.

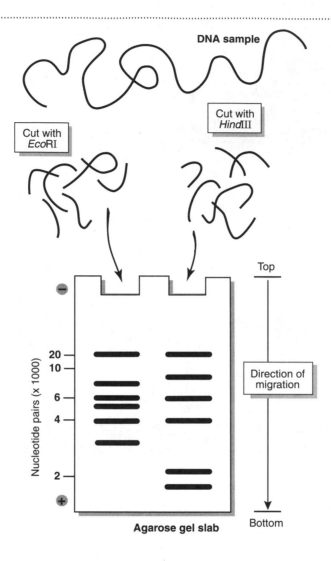

Figure 6-2. Gel electrophoresis of DNA fragments. A DNA sample is cut with restriction enzymes *Eco*RI and *Hind*III. The mixture of DNA fragments obtained from this treatment is placed at the top of an agarose gel slab. Under an electric field, the DNA fragments move through the gel toward the positive electrode (because DNA is negatively charged). DNA fragments in the mixture are separated by size. Small DNA fragments migrate faster than large fragments. Therefore, small fragments are located at the bottom of the gel, and large fragments are located at the top. To permit visualization of the DNA fragments, the gel is soaked in a dye that binds to DNA and fluoresces under ultraviolet light. (Adapted with permission from Alberts B, Bray D, Johnson A et al: *Essential Cell Biology: An Introduction to the Molecular Biology of the Cell*. New York, Garland Publishing, 1998, p. 317.)

    D. Prenatal testing for other genetic diseases. Several single-gene disorders are diagnosed prenatally with DNA analysis, including the following:

        1. Autosomal dominant disorders
            a. Huntington's disease
            b. Myotonic dystrophy
            c. Neurofibromatosis

2. Autosomal recessive disorders
   a. Sickle cell anemia
   b. Cystic fibrosis
   c. Thalassemia α and β
   d. Tay-Sachs disease (GM_2 gangliosidosis)
   e. Phenylketonuria

3. X-linked disorders
   a. Hemophilia A and B
   b. Duchenne type muscular dystrophy

VI. ISOLATING A HUMAN GENE WITH DNA CLONING.

The term "cloning" is confusing because it is used in two ways. First, cloning is making identical copies of a DNA molecule. Second, cloning is isolating one gene from DNA. Isolating, or cloning, one gene from the entire human genome (3×10^9 nucleotide pairs) is a daunting task. Although the cloning method differs from gene to gene, the cloning of **human Factor VIII** illustrates the process. Defects in the gene for Factor VIII cause **hemophilia A.**

A. The first step in cloning human Factor VIII is **constructing a genomic library (Figure 6-5A).** A plasmid vector is a circular DNA molecule that infects and replicates inside a bacterium. Plasmid DNA is combined with human DNA to form a **recombinant plasmid.**

B. The **genomic library is screened (Figure 6-5B)** to identify the bacterial colony that contains the Factor VIII gene.

C. The **gene is amplified (Figure 6-5C)** by culturing the colony in a nutrient broth overnight to produce millions of copies.

D. Another way to eliminate noncoding genes is to **construct a complementary DNA (cDNA) library (Figure 6-6).** Most of the DNA fragments that are recombined with the plasmid vector are either repetitive DNA sequences, introns (noncoding regions), or spacer DNA sequences. These sequences do not code for proteins. Therefore, a large library must be screened to find the gene of interest (e.g., Factor VIII). The main difference between a genomic library and a cDNA library is that a genomic library uses **genomic (chromosomal) DNA,** whereas a cDNA library uses **DNA copied from messenger ribonucleic acid (RNA) [mRNA].** A cDNA library is screened only for the DNA sequences that code for proteins because the DNA used to construct the library is copied from mRNA. The liver is a good candidate organ to construct a cDNA library because it synthesizes large amounts of Factor VIII. **Reverse transcriptase** is the critical enzyme in the creation of a cDNA library because it **produces DNA from an RNA template.**

VII. POLYMERASE CHAIN REACTION (PCR)

A. Mechanism. DNA amplification is one step in cloning the Factor VIII gene with either a genomic library or a cDNA library (see VI C). One method to amplify DNA is to culture bacteria in a nutrient broth overnight. PCR is another method **(Figure 6-7A).** PCR uses **repeated replication cycles** with **specially designed primers, DNA polymerase,** and the deoxyribonucleoside 5′–triphosphates **dATP, dGTP, dCTP, and dTTP.** Some knowledge of the DNA sequence to be amplified is needed to design the primers. Twenty to forty PCR cycles produce millions of copies of the DNA within a few hours.

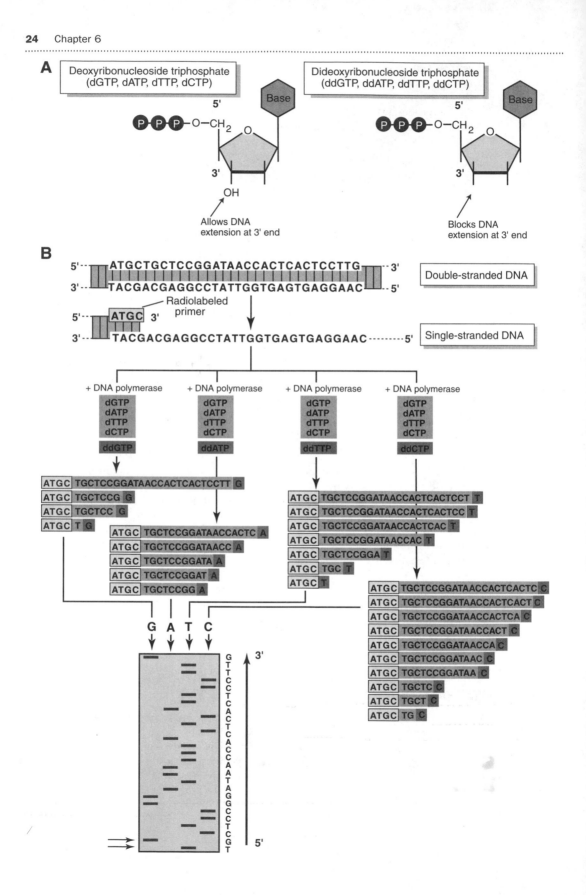

B. PCR and viral detection (Figure 6-7B). After a virus is isolated and its DNA (or RNA) sequence is determined, PCR primers can be designed. Because PCR amplifies even minute amounts of DNA, it is a sensitive method that can detect low levels of viral DNA early in the course of infection.

VIII. PRODUCING A PROTEIN FROM A CLONED GENE. After a gene (e.g., Factor VIII) is cloned with a cloning vector (see VI), the cloned gene is used to produce a protein (i.e., transcribe and translate into the amino acid sequence of a protein). This process **(gene expression)** requires a plasmid (expression) vector.

A. Expression vectors (Figure 6-8A) have the following characteristics:

1. Unlike cloning vectors, they contain gene regulatory and gene promoter DNA sequences that permit expression of a nearby protein-coding DNA sequence.

2. They are used in bacteria, yeast, and mammalian cells.

3. They allow the production of large amounts of any protein, even rare proteins.

4. They are used to produce Factor VIII, human insulin, and human growth hormone.

B. Expression vectors and the nuclear transfer technique (Figure 6-8B)

1. Expression vectors provide another method to produce large amounts of human proteins in the **milk** of large farm animals **(e.g., transgenic sheep, transgenic cows; see IX).**

2. **Human Factor IX,** which is used to treat **hemophilia B,** is produced in the milk of transgenic sheep.

IX. SITE-DIRECTED MUTAGENESIS AND TRANSGENIC ANIMALS (Figure 6-9). The ability to express a cloned gene within a cell opened a new area of medical research. A cloned gene can be mutated at specific sites (site-directed mutagenesis), and the function of the mutant gene can be tested. The cloned gene can be mutated so that as little as one amino acid in the protein is changed **(gene replacement),** or a large deletion can be made so that the protein becomes nonfunctional **(gene knockout).** The ultimate test of the function of the mutant gene is to insert it into an animal genome (e.g., mouse) and observe its effect on the animal. An animal that has a new gene in its genome is called **transgenic. Transgenic mice** are often used in laboratory experiments.

Figure 6-3. Enzymatic method of deoxyribonucleic acid (DNA) sequencing. (A) The biochemical structure of deoxyribonucleoside triphosphates (*dGTP, dATP, dTTP, dCTP*) and dideoxyribonucleoside triphosphates (*ddGTP, ddATP, ddTTP, ddCTP*). The 3′–OH group on the dideoxyribonucleoside triphosphates is missing. (B) Double-stranded DNA is separated into single strands, and one strand is used as a template. A radiolabeled primer (*ATGC*) initiates DNA synthesis. Four reaction mixtures are set up with DNA polymerase, dGTP, dATP, dTTP, dCTP, and either ddGTP, ddATP, ddTTP, or ddCTP. These reactions produce several DNA fragments of different length. The fragments terminate in either G, A, T, or C, depending on which dideoxyribonucleoside triphosphate was present in the reaction mixture. The contents of each reaction mixture are separated by gel electrophoresis, based on DNA fragment size. The gel is exposed to film, and the radiolabeled primer identifies each DNA fragment as a band. The bands are arranged as four parallel columns. Each fragment terminates in either G, A, T, or C. The sequencing gel is read from the bottom of the film. The lowest band (i.e., the shortest DNA fragment; in this case, the T column) is located. After the first nucleotide in the sequence is identified, the next lowest band on the film (in this case, the G column) is located. By repeating this process for all 26 bands, the DNA sequence is constructed in a 5′ → 3′ direction. (Part A adapted with permission from Alberts B, Bray D, Johnson A et al: *Essential Cell Biology: An Introduction to the Molecular Biology of the Cell.* New York, Garland Publishing, 1998, p. 319, Fig. 10-5.)

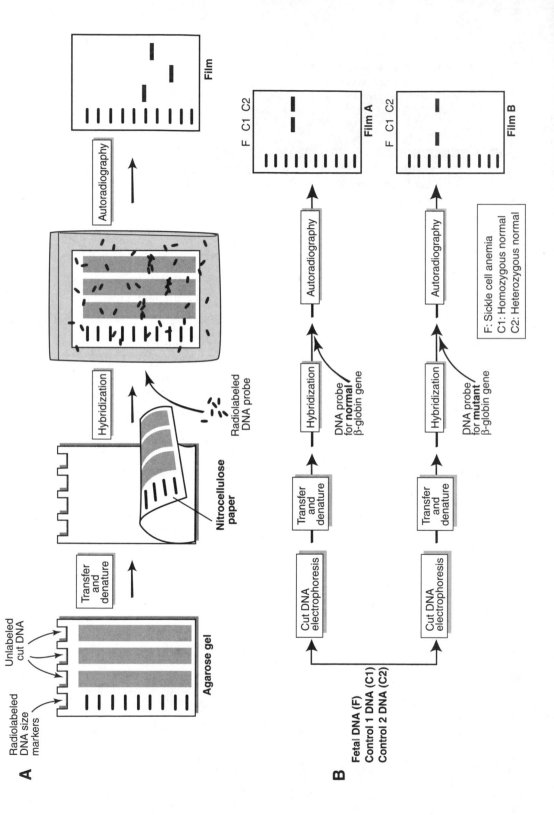

A

Radiolabeled DNA size markers

Unlabeled cut DNA

Agarose gel

Transfer and denature

Nitrocellulose paper

Hybridization

Radiolabeled DNA probe

Autoradiography

Film

B

Fetal DNA (F)
Control 1 DNA (C1)
Control 2 DNA (C2)

Cut DNA electrophoresis

Transfer and denature

Hybridization

DNA probe for **normal** β-globin gene

Autoradiography

F C1 C2

Film A

Cut DNA electrophoresis

Transfer and denature

Hybridization

DNA probe for **mutant** β-globin gene

Autoradiography

F C1 C2

Film B

F: Sickle cell anemia
C1: Homozygous normal
C2: Heterozygous normal

26

Figure 6-4. (A) Southern blotting. Double-stranded deoxyribonucleic acid (DNA) is cut with three restriction enzymes and separated into three lanes with gel electrophoresis. One lane is reserved for radiolabeled DNA size markers. The double-stranded DNA is transferred to nitrocellulose paper under alkaline conditions so that the DNA denatures into single strands. The nitrocellulose paper and the radiolabeled DNA probe are placed in a plastic bag and incubated under conditions that favor hybridization. When the nitrocellulose paper is exposed to photographic film (autoradiography), the radiolabeled probe appears as a series of bands. (B) Prenatal testing for sickle cell anemia. Fetal DNA (F) is obtained from a high-risk fetus and compared with control DNA (C1, C2). The DNA is separated into two samples. After each sample is cut with restriction enzymes, gel electrophoresis is performed. The sample is then transferred to nitrocellulose paper under denaturing conditions. One sample is hybridized with a DNA probe for the normal β-globin gene. The other sample is hybridized with a DNA probe for the mutant β-globin gene. After autoradiography is performed, films A and B are analyzed. Lane F (fetal DNA) has no bands in film A (no normal β-globin gene), but one band in film B (mutant β-globin gene). The fetus is homozygous for the mutant β-globin gene and therefore has sickle cell anemia. Lane C1 (control DNA) has one band in film A, but no bands in film B. This person is homozygous for the normal β-globin gene and therefore is normal. Lane C2 (control DNA) has one band in film A and one band in film B. This person is heterozygous (i.e., has one copy of the normal β-globin gene and one copy of the mutant β-globin gene). This person is normal because sickle cell anemia is an autosomal recessive genetic disease (i.e., it requires two copies of the mutant β-globin gene). (Part A adapted with permission from Alberts B, Bray D, Johnson A et al: *Essential Cell Biology: An Introduction to the Molecular Biology of the Cell.* New York, Garland Publishing, 1998, p. 323.)

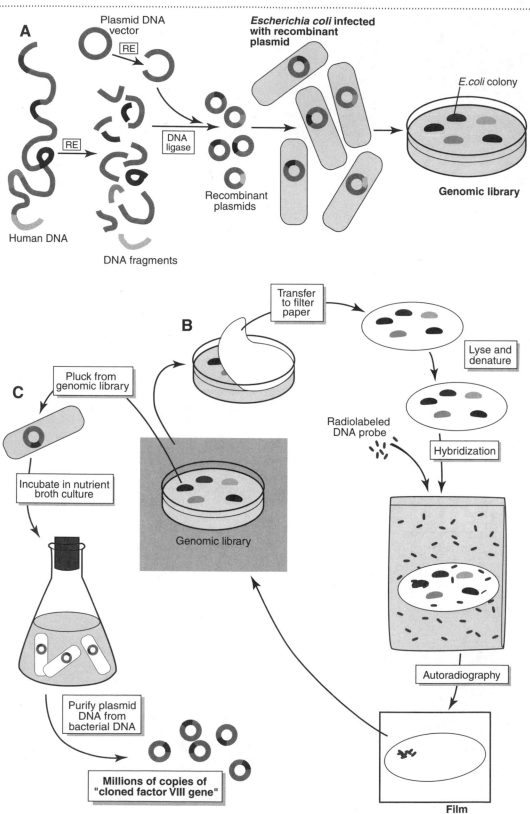

A

Plasmid DNA vector

RE

Escherichia coli infected with recombinant plasmid

E.coli colony

RE

DNA ligase

Recombinant plasmids

Genomic library

Human DNA

DNA fragments

Transfer to filter paper

B

Lyse and denature

Radiolabeled DNA probe

Pluck from genomic library

C

Hybridization

Incubate in nutrient broth culture

Genomic library

Purify plasmid DNA from bacterial DNA

Autoradiography

Millions of copies of "cloned factor VIII gene"

Film

Figure 6-5.   (A) Construction of a genomic library. A restriction enzyme (RE) is used to cut human deoxyribonucleic acid (DNA) into DNA fragments. A plasmid DNA vector is cut with the same restriction enzyme, and the two types of DNA are mixed. Human DNA fragments are inserted into the plasmid DNA and sealed with DNA ligase to form a recombinant plasmid (i.e., DNA from two sources is "recombined"). The recombinant plasmids are mixed with Escherichia coli bacteria and plated on Petri dishes to form bacterial colonies and create a genomic library. (B) Screening the library. The bacterial colonies are transferred to filter paper and lysed, and the DNA is denatured to single strands under alkaline conditions. Because a portion of the amino acid sequence of Factor VIII protein is known, the DNA sequence that codes for these amino acids can be deduced. A DNA probe is made based on the deduced DNA sequence. The radiolabeled DNA probe hybridizes to the DNA strand of a complementary nucleotide sequence (i.e., Factor VIII gene). The filter paper is exposed to photographic film to identify the radiolabeled DNA. (C) Amplification. The corresponding bacterial colony is plucked from the Petri dish and placed in a nutrient broth culture overnight. The recombinant plasmid DNA is separated from the bacterial DNA. Because millions of copies of the recombinant plasmid contain the gene, the Factor VIII gene is now cloned.

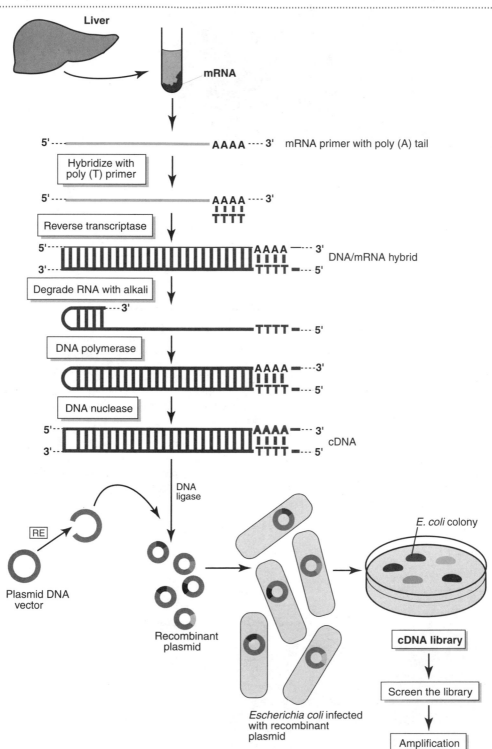

Figure 6-6. Construction of a complementary DNA (cDNA) library. Messenger RNA (mRNA) from the liver is isolated. Copying of only one mRNA into cDNA is shown. The mRNA is hybridized with a poly-T primer, which acts as a primer for reverse transcriptase. Reverse transcriptase copies the mRNA into a cDNA chain to form a DNA/mRNA hybrid. The mRNA is selectively degraded under alkaline conditions. DNA polymerase copies the single strand of DNA into double-stranded DNA, which uses, in this case, the 3′ end of the single-stranded DNA. The 3′ end folds back on itself to form a few chance base pairings. A DNA nuclease cleaves the hairpin loop to form a double-stranded cDNA copy of the original mRNA. The newly formed double-stranded cDNA is inserted into a plasmid vector to create a cDNA library (see Figure 6-5B). *RE* = restriction enzyme.

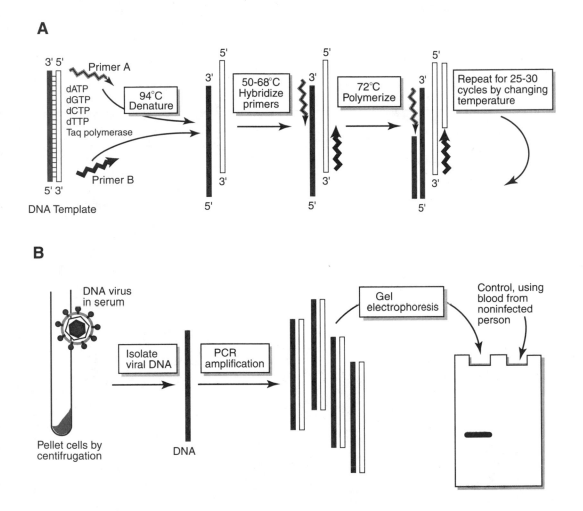

Figure 6-7. (A) Polymerase chain reaction (PCR). A region of double-stranded DNA to be amplified is shown undergoing the PCR. Each cycle of the PCR begins with 94°C heat treatment to separate (denature) the double-stranded DNA into single strands. The DNA primers hybridize to single-stranded DNA and act as the primer for DNA synthesis by DNA (Taq) polymerase, dATP, dGTP, dCTP, and dTTP. Of the DNA put into the original reaction, only the DNA sequence bracketed by the two primers is amplified because no primers are attached anywhere else. This is repeated for 25 to 30 cycles to produce millions of copies of the original region of DNA. (B) PCR and viral detection. A blood sample is taken from a suspect patient, and cells are removed by centrifugation. If even a trace amount of virus is present in the serum, its DNA can be isolated and amplified by PCR. PCR will produce enough DNA so that it can be detected by gel electrophoresis. To detect an RNA virus (e.g., HIV), you must first use reverse transcriptase to convert the RNA to cDNA, and then amplify by PCR. (Part A modified with permission from Jameson JL et al [eds]: *Principles of Molecular Medicine.* Totowa, NJ, Humana Press, 1998, p. 15. Part B reproduced with permission from Alberts B, Bray D, Johnson A et al: *Essential Cell Biology: An Introduction to the Molecular Biology of the Cell.* New York, Garland, 1998, pp. 333–334.)

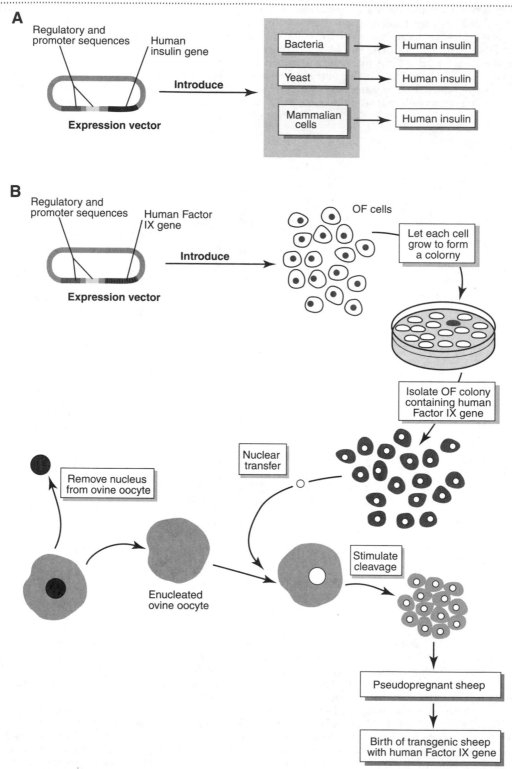

Figure 6-8.   Producing a protein from a cloned gene. (A) An expression vector contains regulatory and promoter DNA sequences that drive the expression of the nearby human insulin gene. The expression vector is introduced into bacteria, yeast, or mammalian cells. The human insulin gene is transcribed and translated into human insulin. This method produces large amounts of human insulin for use by patients with type I and type II diabetes. This method replaced the extraction of insulin from bovine pancreata that were collected from slaughterhouses. (B) Expression vectors and the nuclear transfer technique. Expression vectors contain regulatory and promoter DNA sequences that drive the expression of the nearby human Factor IX gene. The expression vector is introduced into ovine fetal (OF) cells that are cultured to form colonies. The OF colony that contains the human Factor IX gene is isolated. The nucleus of an OF cell that contains the human Factor IX gene is removed and transferred into an enucleated ovine oocyte. The "new" oocyte is stimulated to undergo cleavage. Then it is introduced to a pseudopregnant sheep to produce transgenic sheep. The transgenic sheep have the human Factor IX gene and produce human Factor IX protein in their milk. The nuclear transfer technique causes concern among bioethicists because it leads directly to human cloning. When this technique is perfected, a nucleus from a human cell can be removed, transferred into an enucleated human oocyte, and introduced into a pseudopregnant woman to produce a human clone.

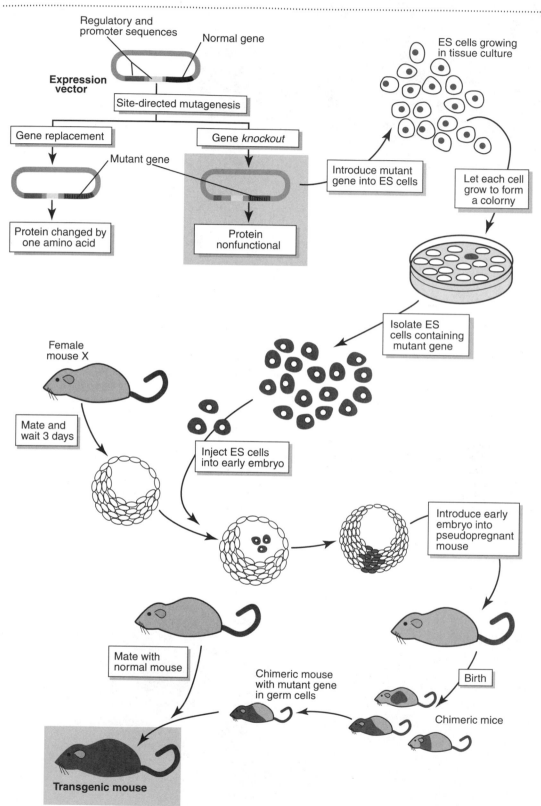

Regulatory and promoter sequences

Normal gene

ES cells growing in tissue culture

Expression vector

Site-directed mutagenesis

Gene replacement

Gene *knockout*

Mutant gene

Introduce mutant gene into ES cells

Let each cell grow to form a colorny

Protein changed by one amino acid

Protein nonfunctional

Isolate ES cells containing mutant gene

Female mouse X

Mate and wait 3 days

Inject ES cells into early embryo

Introduce early embryo into pseudopregnant mouse

Mate with normal mouse

Chimeric mouse with mutant gene in germ cells

Birth

Chimeric mice

Transgenic mouse

Figure 6-9. Site-directed mutagenesis and transgenic animals. An expression vector contains a normal gene that has regulatory and promoter DNA sequences. The mutant gene within the expression vector is introduced into embryonic stem (ES) cells. After the stem cells are cultured, the cells that incorporated the mutant gene (*shaded*) are isolated. These stem cells are injected into an early embryo obtained from a 3-day–pregnant mouse (female mouse X). The embryo contains both cells from female mouse X (*white*) and embryonic stem cells with the mutant gene (*shaded*). Several early embryos are produced and introduced to a pseudopregnant mouse to produce chimeric mice (produced from a mixture of two cell types) [*light and dark shading*]. If a chimeric mouse incorporates the mutant gene into its germ cells, when it mates with a normal mouse, transgenic mice are produced (*dark shading*). A transgenic mouse has one copy of the mutant gene in every cell. (Adapted with permission from Alberts B, Bray D, Johnson A et al: *Essential Cell Biology: An Introduction to the Molecular Biology of the Cell*. New York, Garland, 1998, p. 341.)

7

Control of Gene Expression

I. INTRODUCTION. All human cells contain a set of **housekeeping genes** that produce **housekeeping proteins.** These proteins are used for many functions that are common to all cells (e.g., enzymes for metabolic processes, cytoskeleton proteins, and proteins essential to the endoplasmic reticulum and Golgi complex). Each cell also produces **specialized proteins** (e.g., hepatocytes produce Factor VIII; pancreatic beta cells produce insulin). Because all human cells have identical deoxyribonucleic acid (DNA), the key cell biologic question is: Why do certain cells produce specific proteins? This question is answered by research on the control of gene expression, or **gene regulation.** The most important level of gene regulation is **transcription.**

II. MECHANISM OF GENE REGULATION. Two types of DNA sequences play a role in gene regulation: the **gene promoter DNA sequence** and the **gene regulatory DNA sequence.**

  A. The **gene promoter DNA sequence (Figure 7-1)** has the following characteristics:

    1. It is usually located **near** the gene.

    2. It is located **upstream** of the gene.

    3. It is the site where **ribonucleic acid (RNA) polymerase II** and **transcription factors** assemble so that a gene can be transcribed into messenger RNA (mRNA).

    4. It is located near the **initiation site,** where transcription begins.

    5. It contains a **TATA box** (DNA sequence that is rich in T–A base pairs), **CAAT box,** or **GC box.**

    6. It binds transcription factors that link RNA polymerase II to the promoter to form a **transcription–initiation complex.**

  B. The **gene regulatory (enhancer) DNA sequence (Figure 7-2)** has the following characteristics:

    1. It is usually located **far away** from the gene.

    2. It is located either **upstream** or **downstream** of the gene.

    3. It binds **gene regulatory proteins** that either activate or repress the transcription–initiation complex.

III. STRUCTURE OF TRANSCRIPTION FACTORS AND GENE REGULATORY PROTEINS. Transcription factors and gene regulatory proteins bind to DNA through the interaction of **amino acids** (from the protein) and **nucleotides** (from the DNA).

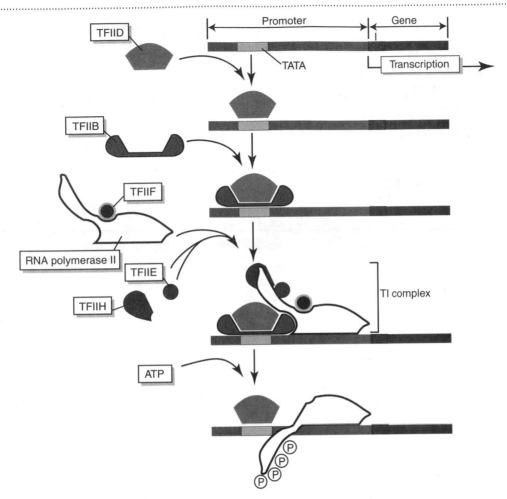

Figure 7-1. The gene promoter and action of transcription factors. The transcription factor TFIID binds to the TATA box, which permits TFIIB binding. The next step involves TFIIE, TFIIH, and TFIIF, and ribonucleic acid (*RNA*) polymerase II engaged to the promoter to form a transcription–initiation (*TI*) complex. TFIIH phosphorylates RNA polymerase II, which is released from the TI complex. RNA polymerase II and the transcription factors are not sufficient to cause transcription within a cell; other factors (gene regulatory proteins) are necessary. *ATP* = adenosine triphosphate. (Adapted with permission from Alberts B, Bray D, Johnson A et al: *Essential Cell Biology: An Introduction to the Molecular Biology of the Cell.* New York, Garland Publishing, 1998, p. 264.)

DNA-binding proteins are classified into **four types:** homeodomain proteins, zinc finger proteins, leucine zipper proteins, and helix–loop–helix proteins.

A. Homeodomain protein (Figure 7-3A)

    1. This protein consists of **three linked alpha helices** (helices 1, 2, and 3). Helices 2 and 3 are arranged in a conspicuous **helix–turn–helix motif.**

    2. A **60 amino acid long region (homeodomain)** within helix 3 binds specifically to DNA segments that contain the sequence **5′-A-T-T-A-3′.**

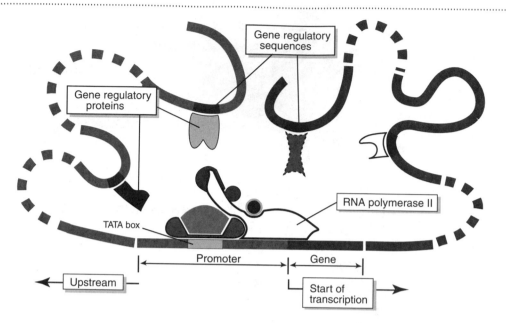

Figure 7-2. The gene regulator and the action of gene regulatory proteins. Gene regulatory sequences bind gene regulatory proteins. These proteins activate or repress the transcription–initiation complex. DNA looping allows gene regulatory proteins that are bound at distant sites to interact with the transcription–initiation complex. *RNA* = ribonucleic acid. (Adapted with permission from Alberts B, Bray D, Johnson A et al: *Essential Cell Biology: An Introduction to the Molecular Biology of the Cell.* New York, Garland Publishing, 1998, p. 268.)

Figure 7-3. Transcription factors and gene regulatory proteins. (*A*) The three-dimensional structure of the Pit-1 homeodomain protein is shown. The 60 amino acid homeodomain of Pit-1 protein is coded for by the *PIT1* gene containing a 180 base pair sequence called the **homeobox sequence**. Pit-1 binding at the transcription–initiation (TI) complex is required for transcription of the genes for growth hormone (*GH*), thyroid-stimulating hormone (*TSH*), and prolactin (*PRL*). A mutation in the gene for Pit-1 will result in the combined deficiency of GH, TSH, and PRL, causing pituitary dwarfism. (*B*) The three-dimensional structure of a specific zinc finger protein (i.e., the glucocorticoid receptor that acts as a gene regulatory protein). The glucocorticoid receptor has a DNA-binding region and a hormone-binding region. In the presence of glucocorticoid hormone, the glucocorticoid receptor will bind to a gene regulatory sequence known as the glucocorticoid response element (GRE), which loops in order to interact with the TI complex and allows the start of gene transcription. (*C*) The three-dimensional structure of a leucine zipper protein (Jun) forming a leucine zipper homodimer (Jun–Jun). *L* = leucine. (*D*) The three-dimensional structure of a helix–loop–helix (HLH) protein forming an HLH homodimer.

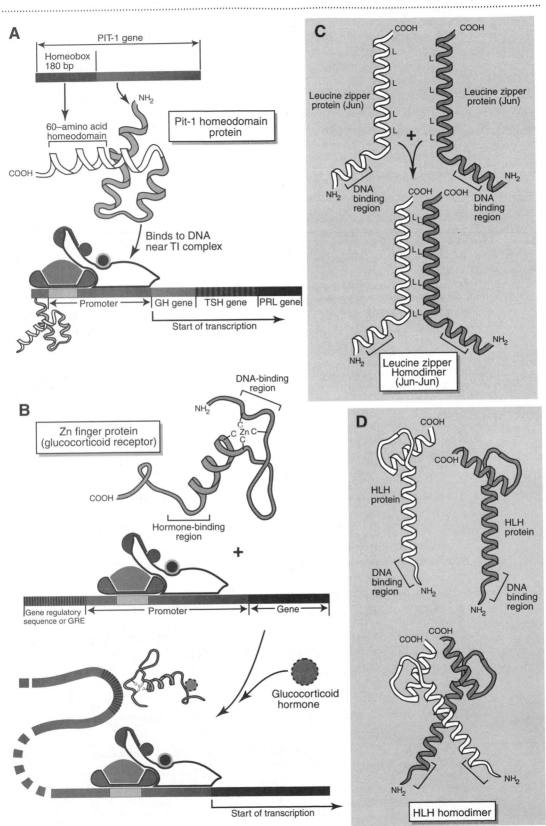

A

PIT-1 gene

Homeobox
180 bp

60–amino acid
homeodomain

COOH

NH₂

Pit-1 homeodomain
protein

Binds to DNA
near TI complex

Promoter | GH gene | TSH gene | PRL gene

Start of transcription

B

Zn finger protein
(glucocorticoid receptor)

NH₂

DNA-binding
region

C C
C Zn C
C

COOH

Hormone-binding
region

+

Gene regulatory
sequence or GRE | Promoter | Gene

Glucocorticoid
hormone

Start of transcription

C

COOH   COOH

L   L
L   L
L   L
L   L
L   L

Leucine zipper
protein (Jun)

Leucine zipper
protein (Jun)

NH₂   DNA
binding
region

+

DNA
binding   NH₂
region

COOH COOH

L L
L L
L L
L L
L L

NH₂

NH₂

Leucine zipper
Homodimer
(Jun-Jun)

D

COOH

COOH

HLH
protein

HLH
protein

DNA
binding
region   NH₂

DNA
binding
region
NH₂

COOH COOH

NH₂   NH₂

HLH homodimer

3. Specific **examples** of homeodomain proteins are:
   a. **Octanucleotide binding protein-1 (OCT-1),** which regulates the histone gene H2B, the thymidine kinase gene, and snRNP genes
   b. **Octanucleotide binding protein-2 (OCT-2),** which regulates various immuno-globulin genes
   c. **Pituitary specific factor-1 (Pit-1),** which regulates the growth hormone gene, the thyroid-stimulated hormone gene, and the prolactin gene.

B. **Zinc finger protein (see Figure 7-3B)**

   1. It has **one alpha helix.**

   2. It contains **one zinc atom** bound to **four cysteine amino acids.**

   3. It contains a **hormone-binding region.**

   4. A **70 amino acid long region** near the zinc atom binds specifically to DNA segments.

   5. Specific **examples** of zinc finger proteins are:
      a. **Transcription factor IIIA (TFIIIA),** which engages RNA polymerase II to the gene promoter
      b. **Sp1** (first described for its action on the SV40 promoter), which engages RNA polymerase II to the gene promoter by binding to the GC box
      c. **Glucocorticoid receptor, estrogen receptor, progesterone receptor, thyroid hormone receptor (erbA), retinoic acid receptor,** and the **vitamin D3 receptor**

C. **Leucine zipper protein (see Figure 7-3C)**

   1. It consists of an **alpha helix** that contains a region in which **every seventh amino acid is leucine,** which has the effect of lining up all the leucine residues on one side of the alpha helix.

   2. The leucine residues allow for **dimerization** of the two leucine zipper proteins and formation of a **Y- shaped dimer.**

   3. Dimerization may occur between two of the same proteins (**homodimers,** e.g., Jun–Jun) or two different proteins (**heterodimers,** e.g., Fos–Jun).

   4. It contains a **20 amino acid long region** that binds specifically to DNA segments.

   5. Specific **examples** of leucine zipper proteins are:
      a. **CCAAT/enhancer binding protein (C/EBP),** which regulates the albumin gene and the α1-antitrypsin gene
      b. **Cyclic AMP response element binding protein (CREB),** which regulates the somatostatin gene and the proenkephalin gene
      c. **Finkel osteogenic sarcoma virus (Fos) protein,** a product of the c-*fos* proto-oncogene, which regulates various genes involved in the cell cycle and cell transformation
      d. **Jun protein,** a product of the c-*jun* proto-oncogene, which regulates various genes involved in the cell cycle and cell transformation

D. **Helix–loop–helix protein (HLH) [Figure 7-3D]**

   1. It consists of a short alpha helix connected by a loop to a longer alpha helix.

   2. The loop allow for **dimerization** of two HLH proteins and formation of a **Y-shaped dimer.**

   3. Dimerization may occur between two of the same proteins (**homodimers**) or two different proteins (**heterodimers**).

4. Specific **examples** of HLH proteins are:
   a. **MyoD protein,** which regulates various genes involved in muscle development
   b. **Myc protein,** a product of the **c-myc protooncogene,** which regulates various genes involved in the cell cycle.

IV. CLINICAL CONSIDERATION: GROWTH HORMONE DEFICIENCY AND PIT-1 TRANSCRIPTION FACTOR (see Figure 7-3A). Approximately 1 of every 10,000 newborns has a growth hormone (GH) deficiency that causes **pituitary dwarfism.** Some of these infants are also deficient in thyroid-stimulating hormone (TSH) and prolactin (PRL).

A. The combined deficiency of GH, TSH, and PRL is caused by a **mutation in the gene** that encodes for a transcription factor **(Pit-1).** Pit-1 is a homeodomain protein that is required for GH, TSH, and PRL transcription.

B. Genetic screening for mutations in the *PIT1* gene permits presymptomatic diagnosis.

C. Patients are given injections of GH that is produced with recombinant DNA technology.

V. THE *lac* OPERON. An operon is a set of coordinately controlled genes adjacent to one another in the genome. The details of gene regulation were first discovered by Drs. Jacob and Monod in *E. coli* bacteria and the *lac* operon.

A. The *lac* operon consists of **three genes:**

   1. The *lac* Z gene encodes **β-galactosidase,** which splits lactose into glucose and galactose.

   2. The *lac* Y gene encodes **lactose permease,** which pumps lactose into the cell.

   3. The *lac* A gene encodes **thiogalactosidase transacetylase,** the function of which is not well understood.

B. The enzyme β-galactosidase is easily assayed using a colorless compound commonly called **X-gal,** which is hydrolyzed by β-galactosidase into a blue product, providing an easy colormetric assay.

C. *E. coli* grown in **glucose+ medium** express **low levels of the *lac* Z and *lac* Y genes.** *E. coli* switched to a **lactose+ medium** express **high levels of the *lac* Z and *lac* Y genes.** This led to the concept that lactose was an **inducer** of gene expression.

D. *E. coli* mutants, when isolated and grown in glucose+ medium, express high levels of the *lac* Z and *lac* Y genes. These mutants are called **constitutive** because they fail to repress the *lac* operon, and thereby continuously (or constitutively) express high levels of the *lac* Z and *lac* Y genes even in the presence of glucose. These mutations were mapped to a region on the *E. coli* chromosome to the left of the *lac* Z gene and were named *lac* I genes. This discovery led to the concept that the protein encoded by the *lac* I gene was a repressor of gene expression. This protein is called the *lac* repressor.

VI. SUMMARY. Each cell produces a specialized protein because it contains a **unique combination of transcription factors and gene regulatory proteins** to stimulate transcription of that gene. Hepatocytes and pancreatic beta cells each have a unique combination of transcription factors and gene regulatory proteins that stimulates the transcription of the Factor VIII gene and the insulin gene, respectively.

8

Protein Synthesis

I. TRANSCRIPTION (**Figure 8-1**) has the following characteristics:

   A. It is the mechanism by which cells copy **deoxyribonucleic acid (DNA)** to **ribonucleic acid (RNA).**

   B. It occurs in the nucleus.

   C. It is performed by one of three enzymes:

   1. **RNA polymerase I,** which produces ribosomal RNA (rRNA).

   2. **RNA polymerase II,** which produces **messenger RNA (mRNA)** and **small nuclear ribonucleic proteins (snRNPs).**

   3. **RNA polymerase III, which** produces **transfer RNA (tRNA)** and **5S rRNA.**

   D. RNA polymerases copy a DNA template strand in the **3′ to 5′** direction, which produces an RNA transcript in the **5′ to 3′** direction.

II. CONVERTING AN RNA TRANSCRIPT TO mRNA (**Figure 8-2**). A cell that is involved in protein synthesis uses RNA polymerase II to transcribe a protein-coding gene into an **RNA transcript** that is further processed into mRNA. This processing involves:

   A. RNA capping (addition of a **methylated guanine nucleotide** to the **5′ end** of the RNA transcript), which increases the stability of mRNA and aids its export from the nucleus.

   B. RNA polyadenylation [addition of repeated adenine nucleotides (**poly-A tail**) to the 3′ end of the RNA transcript], which increases the stability of mRNA and aids its export from the nucleus.

   C. RNA splicing

   1. RNA splicing is a process that **removes all introns** and **joins all exons** within the RNA transcript.

   2. This splicing is performed by **snRNPs** that are a complex of RNA and protein called a **spliceosome.** The RNA portion hybridizes to a nucleotide sequence that marks the intron site. The protein portion removes the intron and rejoins the RNA transcript.

   3. RNA splicing produces **mRNA** that leaves the nucleus to undergo translation in the cytoplasm.

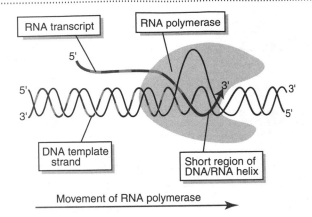

RNA transcript

RNA polymerase

5′

5′
3′

3′

3′
5′

DNA template
strand

Short region of
DNA/RNA helix

Movement of RNA polymerase

Figure 8-1. Transcription. One of the strands of the DNA double helix acts as a deoxyribonucleic acid (*DNA*) template strand to produce a ribonucleic acid (*RNA*) transcript. RNA polymerase copies the DNA template strand in a 3′ to 5′ direction to produce a RNA transcript in the 5′ to 3′ direction. Short regions of the DNA/RNA helix are transiently produced. The RNA transcript is single-stranded. The nucleotides that synthesize RNA are the ribonucleoside triphosphates (ATP, UTP, GTP, and CTP). (Reprinted with permission from Alberts B, Bray D, Johnson A et al: *Essential Cell Biology: An Introduction to the Molecular Biology of the Cell.* New York, Garland, 1998, p. 215.)

III. TRANSLATION (Figures 8-3 and 8-4) has the following characteristics:

A. It is the mechanism by which the **mRNA nucleotide sequence** is translated into the **amino acid sequence** of a protein.

B. It occurs in the **cytoplasm** using **rough endoplasmic reticulum (rER)** and **polyribosomes.**

C. It decodes a set of **three nucleotides (codon)** into **one amino acid** (e.g., GCA codes for alanine; UAC codes for tyrosine). The codon is **redundant** (i.e., more than one codon specifies one amino acid (e.g., GCA, GCC, GCG, and GCU all specify alanine; UAC and UAU both specify tyrosine).

D. It uses **tRNA,** which has two important binding sites. The first site **(anticodon)** binds to the complementary codon on the mRNA. The second site binds a particular amino acid.

E. It uses the enzyme **aminoacyl-tRNA synthetase,** which links an amino acid to tRNA. Each amino acid has a specific aminoacyl-tRNA synthetase. Because there are 20 different amino acids, there are 20 different aminoacyl-tRNA synthetase enzymes.

F. It uses the enzyme **peptidyl transferase,** which helps to form the peptide bond between amino acids.

G. It requires an organelle **(ribosome),** which is a complex that contains at lease 50 **ribosomal proteins** and **rRNA.** Large ribosome assemblies are called **polyribosomes,** or **polysomes.**

H. The ribosome moves along the mRNA in a **5′ to 3′ direction.** The **NH$_2$-terminal end** of a protein is synthesized **first,** and the **COOH-terminal end** is synthesized **last.**

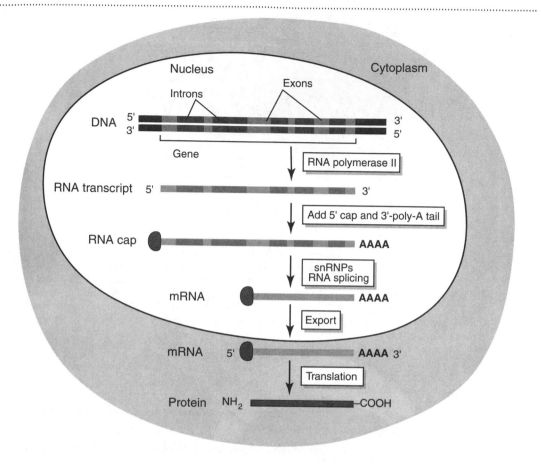

Figure 8-2. Transcription and processing of ribonucleic acid *(RNA)* into messenger RNA *(mRNA)*. All eucaryotic genes contain noncoding regions (introns) separated by coding regions (exons). During transcription, RNA polymerase II transcribes both intron and exon sequences into an RNA transcript. A 5′-cap and a 3′-poly-A tail are added. The introns are spliced out of the RNA transcript by small nuclear ribonucleoprotein particles *(snRNPs)* [the complex is a splisosome] so that all of the exons are joined in sequence. The mRNA, with the 5′-cap and the 3′-poly-A tail, exits the nucleus through the nuclear pore complex and enters the cytoplasm, where it is translated into protein. *DNA* = deoxyribonucleic acid. (Reprinted with permission from Alberts B, Bray D, Johnson A et al: *Essential Cell Biology: An Introduction to the Molecular Biology of the Cell.* New York, Garland, 1998, p. 223.)

Figure 8-3. Translation. Three amino acids are linked (amino acids 1, 2, and 3). Translation is a three-step process that is repeated many times during protein synthesis. The enzyme aminoacyl-transfer ribonucleic acid *(tRNA)* synthetase links a specific amino acid with its specific tRNA. In step 1, the tRNA and amino acid complex 4 bind to site A on the ribosome. The ribosome moves along the messenger RNA *(mRNA)* in a 5′ to 3′ direction. In step 2, the enzyme peptidyl transferase forms a peptide bond between amino acids 3 and 4. The small subunit of the ribosome reconfigures and leaves site A vacant. In step 3, the used tRNA 3 is ejected. The ribosome is then ready for tRNA and amino acid complex 5. (Reprinted with permission from Alberts B, Bray D, Johnson A et al: *Essential Cell Biology: An Introduction to the Molecular Biology of the Cell.* New York, Garland, 1998, p. 230.)

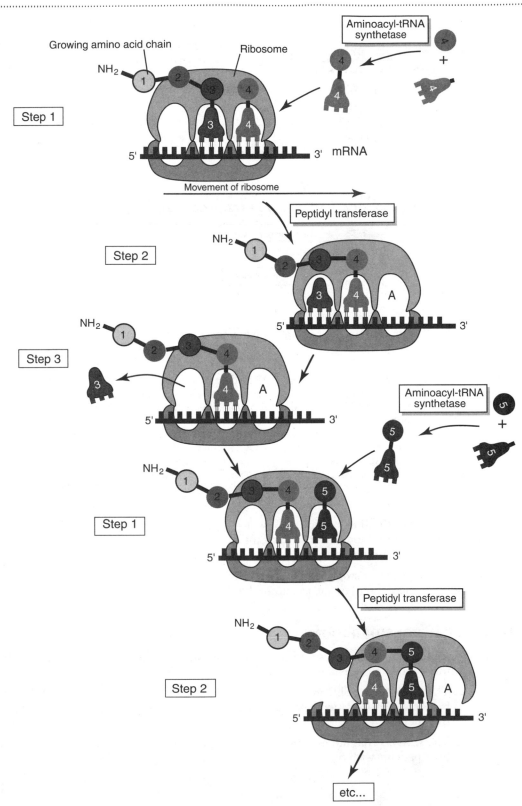

Step 1

Growing amino acid chain

Ribosome

Aminoacyl-tRNA synthetase

NH_2

Movement of ribosome

5'   3'   mRNA

Peptidyl transferase

Step 2

NH_2

A

Step 3

NH_2

5'   3'

Aminoacyl-tRNA synthetase

Step 1

NH_2

5'   3'

Peptidyl transferase

Step 2

NH_2

5'   3'

A

etc...

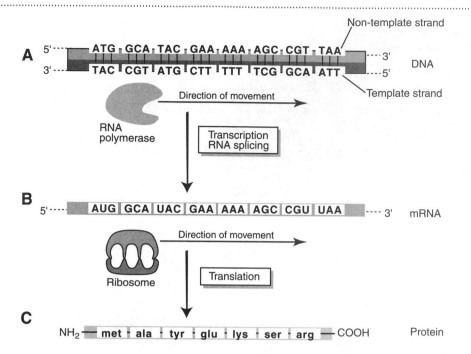

Figure 8-4. Transcription through translation. (A) The deoxyribonucleic acid (*DNA*) sequence, with template and nontemplate strands. Ribonucleic acid (*RNA*) polymerase copies the template strand in the 3′ to 5′ direction and produces messenger RNA (*mRNA*) in the 5′ to 3′ direction. In mRNA, uracil (U) pairs with adenine (A). (B) The mRNA nucleotide sequence, which indicates the start codon (*AUG*), codons for each amino acid, and the stop codon (*UAA*). The ribosome reads the mRNA in a 5′ to 3′ direction. The NH_2-terminal end of the protein is synthesized first, and the COOH-terminal end is synthesized last. (C) The amino acid sequence of the protein. AUG = methionine (*met*); GCA = alanine (*ala*); UAC = tyrosine (*tyr*); GAA = glutamic acid (*glu*); AAA = lysine (*lys*); AGC = serine (*ser*); CGU = arginine (*arg*).

I. It begins with the **start codon AUG,** which codes for **methionine.** All newly synthesized proteins have methionine as their first (or NH_2-terminal) amino acid. Methionine is usually removed later by a protease.

J. It terminates at the **stop codon (UAA,UAG,UGA).** The stop codon binds **release factors** that cause the ribosome to release the protein into the cytoplasm.

IV. CLINICAL CONSIDERATIONS

A. Systemic lupus erythematosus (SLE) is a chronic autoimmune disease that causes rashes, arthritis, and kidney disease.

1. The symptoms of SLE are due to inflammation caused by the deposition of the antibody complexes. Patients produce autoantibodies, frequently against components of the nucleus.

2. The snRNPs that are used in RNA splicing were first characterized with antibodies from patients with SLE.

B. β° **thalassemia** is a genetic disease whereby the affected individual is unable to synthesize the β-globin protein, and thus produces far too little hemoglobin. This causes severe anemia in the affected individual.

   1. Adult hemoglobin consists of two α-**globin proteins** and two β-**globin proteins.** The β-globin gene has three exons and two introns. The introns contain a **G-T sequence** that is responsible for the occurrence of correct RNA splicing and the formation of normal β-globin mRNA.

   2. In β° thalassemia, the G-T sequence is mutated to A-T such that correct RNA splicing does NOT occur, and the defective β-globin mRNA cannot be translated into β-globin protein.

9

The Nucleolus

I. ORGANIZATION OF THE NUCLEOLUS (Figure 9-1)

A. The nucleolus contains approximately **200 copies of ribosomal ribonucleic acid (rRNA) genes** per haploid genome.

B. The 200 copies of rRNA genes are arranged in clusters called the **nucleolar organizer** on **chromosomes 13, 14, 15, 21, and 22.**

C. The rRNA genes within the nucleolar organizer are arranged in a **tandem series.**

D. **RNA polymerase I** transcribes the rRNA genes to form **45S RNA.**

E. Another set of rRNA genes is located outside the nucleolus. **RNA polymerase III** transcribes these genes to form **5S RNA.**

II. ASSEMBLY OF THE RIBOSOME (Figure 9-2)

A. The 45S RNA joins 5S RNA, ribosomal protein, RNA- binding proteins (e.g., nucleolin), and small ribonuclear proteins (snRNPs) to form a large complex.

B. The 45S RNA in the large complex is cut into **5.8S RNA, 18S RNA, and 28S RNA.** The large complex then splits into two subunits:

    1. The **40S subunit,** which contains 18S RNA.

    2. The **60S subunit,** which contains 5S RNA, 5.8S RNA, and 28S RNA.

C. These subunits are transported through nuclear pores into the cytoplasm, where they are assembled into **ribosomes.**

III. ULTRASTRUCTURE OF THE NUCLEOLUS (see Figure 9-2)

A. The **fibrillar center** is pale-staining and contains **transcriptionally inactive DNA.**

B. The **dense fibrillar component** is dense-staining and contains **transcriptionally active DNA, RNA polymerase I, and 45S RNA.**

C. The **granular component** contains maturing ribosomal precursors, including **45S RNA, 5S RNA, ribosomal proteins, RNA-binding proteins,** and **snRNPs.**

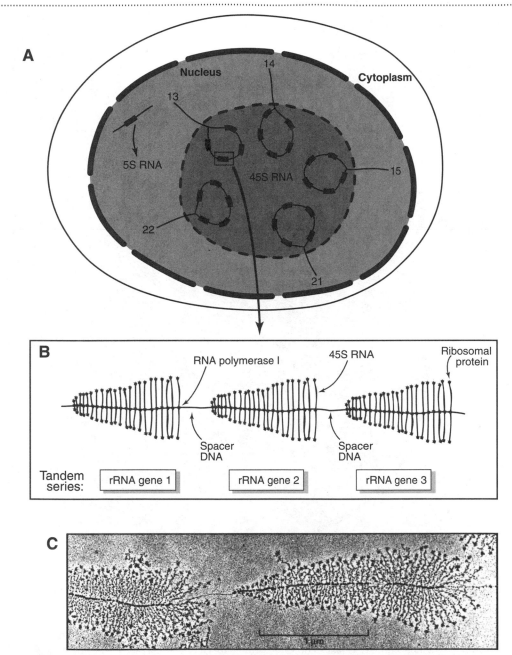

Figure 9-1. Organization of the nucleolus. (A) The non–membrane-bound nucleolus (dotted lines) contains DNA loops from chromosomes 13, 14, 15, 21, and 22. The rRNA genes are organized on these DNA loops as nucleolar organizers (small box). The 5S RNA is transcribed by genes that are located outside the nucleolus. (B) The nucleolar organizer. Three rRNA genes are arranged in a tandem series and separated by spacer DNA. During transcription of rRNA genes, a Christmas tree pattern is seen ultrastructurally. A particle that corresponds to RNA polymerase I, 45S RNA segments of varying lengths, and a particle that corresponds to ribosomal proteins that are involved in early packaging are shown. (C) Electron micrograph of an rRNA gene that is undergoing transcription and shows the Christmas tree pattern. (Courtesy of Ulrich Scheer. Reprinted with permission from Alberts B, Bray D, Johnson A et al: *Essential Cell Biology: An Introduction to the Molecular Biology of the Cell*. New York, Garland, 1998.)

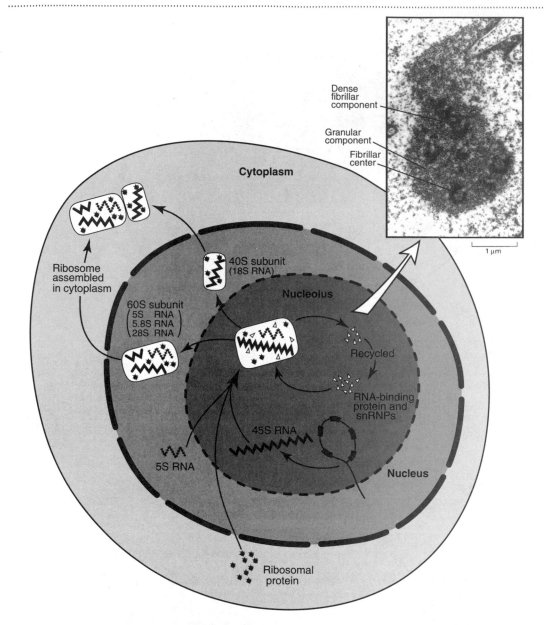

Figure 9-2. Assembly of the ribosome. The 45S recombinant ribonucleic acid (rRNA) joins 5S RNA, ribosomal proteins, RNA-binding proteins (e.g., nucleolin), and small ribonucleoprotein particles (snRNPs) to form a large complex. This complex splits into 40S and 60S subunits. The subunits are transported into the cytoplasm individually and assembled into ribosomes. *Inset:* Electron micrograph of the nucleolus, including the dense fibrillar component, granular component, and fibrillar center. (Reprinted with permission from E.G. Jordan and J. McGovern. Reprinted with permission from Alberts B, Bray D, Johnson A et al: *Essential Cell Biology: An Introduction to the Molecular Biology of the Cell.* New York, Garland, 1998, pp 916- 917.)

10

Mutations of the DNA Sequence

I. SILENT MUTATIONS (Figure 10-1) occur when a change in the nucleotides alters the codon, but no phenotypic change is seen in the individual. These mutations **produce functional proteins** and may occur in:

A. **Spacer DNA,** in which no genes or proteins are altered (see Figure 10-1A).

B. **Introns,** in which the protein is not altered because introns are spliced out as messenger ribonucleic acid (mRNA) is made (see Figure 10-1B). A mutation that occurs near a splice site may alter the protein (see VI).

C. The **third nucleotide of the codon** (see Figure 10-1C). This nucleotide is often mutated without changing the amino acid for which it codes. This situation, called **third nucleotide (base) redundancy,** occurs because one amino acid has several codons.

II. MISSENSE MUTATIONS (Figure 10-2A) occur when a change in a single nucleotide alters the codon so that **one amino acid in a protein replaces another amino acid.** These mutations **produce proteins with a compensated function** if they occur at an active or catalytic site or if they alter the three-dimensional structure of the protein.

III. NONSENSE MUTATIONS (see Figure 10-2B) occur when a change in a single nucleotide alters the codon and produces a **premature stop codon.** These mutations **produce nonfunctional (truncated) proteins** that are unstable and readily degraded.

IV. FRAMESHIFT MUTATIONS (see Figure 10-2C) occur when a deletion or an insertion of a single nucleotide alters the codon and **shifts the reading frame.** These mutations **produce nonfunctional ("garbled") proteins** because they change all of the amino acids that occur after the deletion or insertion.

V. TRANSLOCATION MUTATIONS (Figure 10-3A) occur when a **section of a gene moves** from its original location to another location, either on the same chromosome or on a different chromosome. These mutations may **produce no protein.**

VI. RNA SPLICING MUTATIONS (see Figure 10-3B) occur when a change in the nucleotide at the 5′- or 3′- end of an intron alters the codon and **changes a splice site in the RNA transcript.** These mutations **produce no protein** because the mRNA is unstable and rapidly degraded.

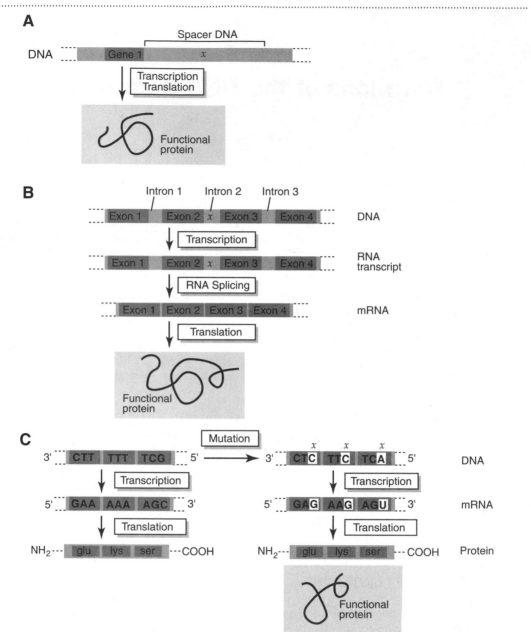

Figure 10-1.   Silent mutation within (A) the spacer deoxyribonucleic acid (DNA), (B) the intron, or (C) the third nucleotide of the codon. RNA = ribonucleic acid; mRNA = messenger RNA. x = cite of mutation.

Figure 10-2.   (A) Missense, (B) nonsense, and (C) frameshift mutations. DNA = deoxyribonucleic acid; mRNA = messenger ribonucleic acid.

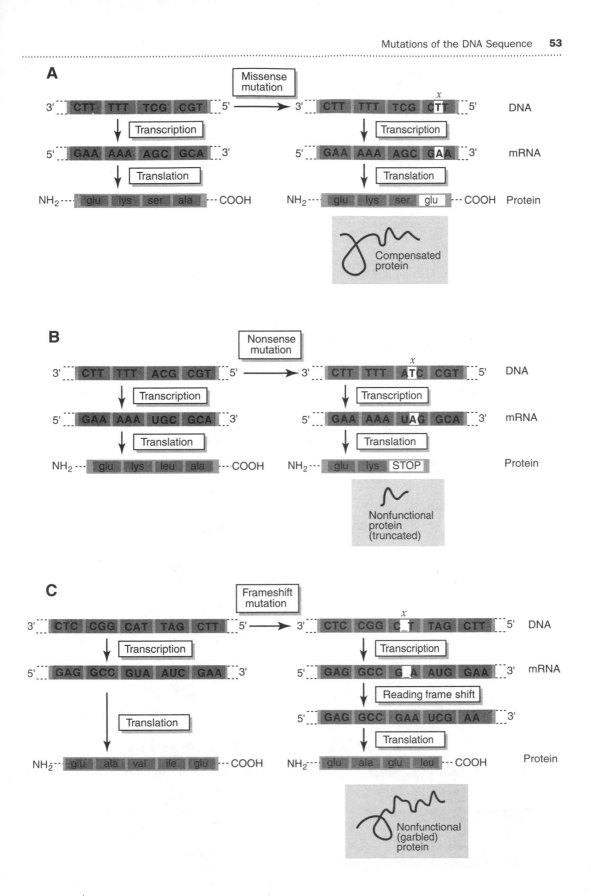

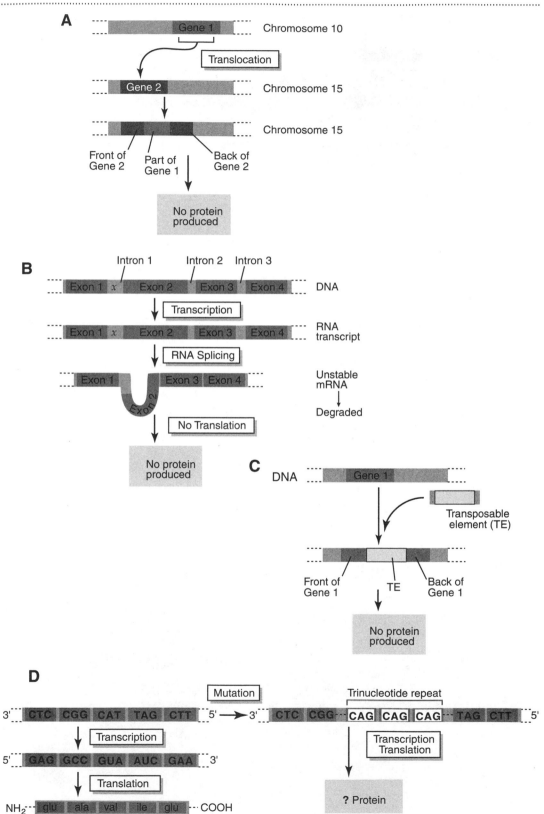

VII. TRANSPOSABLE ELEMENT MUTATIONS (see Figure 10-3C) occur when a transposable element (see Chapter 4) alters the codon and disrupts a gene. These mutations produce no protein because they disrupt the gene. Although transposition is common in the human genome, it rarely disrupts a gene.

VIII. TRINUCLEOTIDE REPEAT MUTATIONS (see Figure 10-3D) occur when a three-nucleotide sequence (CAG, CGG, or CTG) is abnormally repeated, sometimes as many as 200 to 1000 times. These mutations cause Kennedy's syndrome, fragile X syndrome, myotonic dystrophy, and Huntington's disease.

Figure 10-3. (*A*) Translocation mutation. (*B*) Ribonucleic acid (RNA) splicing mutation. (*C*) Transposable element mutation. (*D*) Trinucleotide repeat mutation. *DNA* = deoxyribonucleic acid; *mRNA* = messenger ribonucleic acid.

11

Molecular Genetics

I. POLYMORPHISMS

A. Definitions

1. A **gene** is a hereditary factor that interacts with the environment to produce a trait.

2. An **allele** is an alternative version of a gene or deoxyribonucleic acid (DNA) segment.

3. A **locus** is the location of a gene or DNA segment on a chromosome. Because human chromosomes are paired, humans have two alleles at each locus.

4. A **polymorphism** is the occurrence of two or more alleles at a specific locus in frequencies greater than can be explained by mutations alone. Polymorphisms are common in **noncoding regions of DNA (introns).** A polymorphism is not a mutation that causes a genetic disease; however, a polymorphism can be used as a **genetic marker** for a gene (e.g., the dystrophin gene in Duchenne type muscular dystrophy) when the polymorphism and the dystrophin gene are closely linked.

B. Types of polymorphisms (Figure 11-1)

1. Restriction fragment length polymorphisms (RFLPs)
   a. RFLPs either **create or destroy a restriction enzyme site.**
   b. RFLPs are abundant throughout the human genome and have been widely used in **gene linkage** and **gene mapping** studies.

2. Variable number of tandem repeats (VNTRs)
   a. VNTRs **leave the restriction enzyme site intact, but alter the length of the restriction enzyme fragments** as determined by the number of tandem repeats.
   b. VNTRs are DNA sequences (11–60 base pairs long) that are repeated in tandem in the human genome between restriction enzyme sites a variable number of times.
   c. Because VNTRs are extremely polymorphic, two unrelated people cannot exhibit the same genotype.
   d. VNTRs are used in **DNA fingerprinting and forensic medicine** to establish paternity, zygosity, or identity from a blood, semen, or other DNA sample.

II. LINKAGE (COINHERITANCE) [Figure 11-2]

A. Linkage is the closeness of two or more loci on a chromosome. The loci sort together during **meiosis.**

B. Linkage refers to **loci, not alleles.**

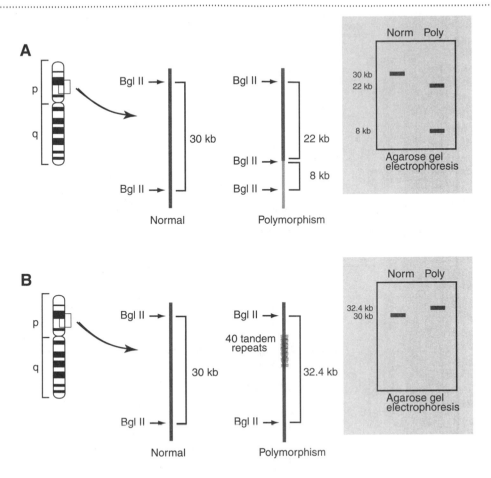

Figure 11-1.   (A) RFLPs. At a certain locus on a chromosome, two Bgl II restriction enzyme sites produce a 30-kb fragment that is observable with agarose gel electrophoresis. A third Bgl II restriction enzyme site produces a 22-kb fragment and an 8-kb fragment. (B) VNTRs. At a certain locus on a chromosome, two Bgl II restriction enzyme sites produce a 30-kb fragment that is observable with agarose gel electrophoresis. The VNTR has 40 tandem repeats of 60 base pairs (40 × 60 = 2400 base pairs) inserted to produce a 32.4-kb fragment. RFLPs and VNTRs that are closely linked to a certain gene (e.g., the dystrophin gene) provide a genetic marker for the gene and allow the inheritance of a mutation to be traced in an affected family. VNTRs are usually better markers than RFLPs.

C. Linkage occurs because crossover (the exchange of DNA between homologous chromosomes that occurs in meiosis I during chiasmata formation) rarely occurs between loci that are close together.

D. It can be measured **only in family studies (pedigrees)** because meiosis that is required to demonstrate linkage occurs only during gametogenesis. Consequently, only family members can be used to determine linkage.

E. Table 11-1 shows the units of measurement of linkage.

   1. Centimorgans (cM)

   2. Recombination fraction (θ)

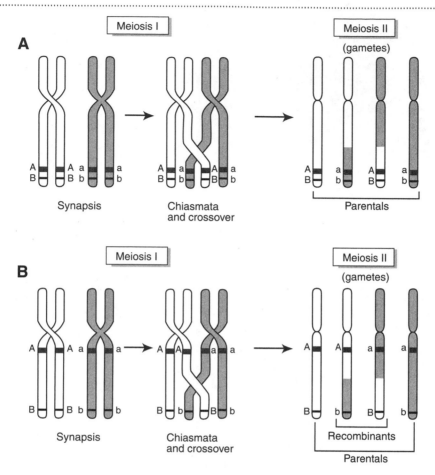

Figure 11-2. (A) High linkage (0 cM, 0.00 θ = 0.0%, LOD score ≥ ⁺3). In meiosis I, two homologous chromosomes undergo synapsis (pairing of homologous chromosomes), chiasmata, and crossover. In this case, the loci *(bars)* are close together, and the alleles *(A, B, a, and b)* are not separated by crossover. In meiosis II, the gametes that are formed have the same allele pattern as the parents *(parentals)*. (B) No linkage (50 cM, 0.50 θ = 50%, LOD score ≤ ⁻2. In meiosis I, two homologous chromosomes undergo synapsis (pairing of homologous chromosomes), chiasmata, and crossover. In this case, the loci *(bars)* are far apart, and the alleles *(A, B, a, and b)* are separated by crossover. In meiosis II, the gametes that are formed have the same allele pattern as the parents *(parentals)* as well as alleles in a different pattern *(recombinants)*.

> **3. Logarithm of the odds (LOD) score:** Because one pedigree usually does not provide convincing evidence of linkage, data from a number of pedigrees are combined and expressed as a LOD score.
>
> **F.** **Adult polycystic kidney disease (APKD)** is a clinical example of linkage **(Figure 11-3).**

III. POPULATION GENETICS

> **A.** According to the **Hardy-Weinberg (genetic) equilibrium theory, allele frequency** and **genotype frequency** in a population remain **constant** from generation to generation as long as no outside influence affects the frequencies (e.g., no mutations occur, no selection occurs, mating is random). This theorem is fundamental to the study of population genetics.

Table 11-1.
Measurements of Linkage

Linkage		Centimorgans (cM)	Recombination Fraction θ %Recombination (%)	LOD Score
High		0	0.00 θ = 0.0%*	≥ ⁺3
Intermediate		1 5 10	0.01 θ = 1.0%⁺ 0.05 θ = 5.0%ǂ 0.10 θ = 10%§	≥ ⁺3
None		50	0.50 θ = 50%‖	≤ ⁻2

*0% chance of crossover between loci.
⁺ 1% chance of crossover between loci.
ǂ 5% chance of crossover between loci.
§ 10% chance of crossover between loci.
‖ 50% chance of crossover between loci.

B. **The Hardy-Weinberg law** states that for a locus with two alleles **(S and s)** with frequencies of **p** and **q,** respectively, the genotype frequencies are:

1. SS = p^2

2. Ss = 2pq

3. ss = q^2

C. Examples of the Hardy-Weinberg law using sickle cell anemia

1. Example 1

    a. **Question:** What is the genotype frequency of homozygous normal black Americans for sickle cell anemia if the S and s allele frequencies are p = 0.96 and q = 0.04, respectively?

    b. **Solution:** Homozygous normal individuals have a genotype of SS. The genotype frequency of SS = p^2. Therefore, 0.96^2 = 0.9216, or 92.16%. Dividing 100/92.16 = 1.08. Therefore, the frequency of normal individuals who are homozygous for sickle cell anemia is 92.16%, or 1 of 1.08 black Americans.

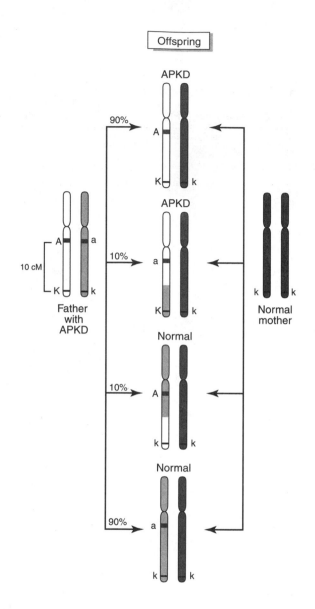

Figure 11-3. Clinical example of linkage: adult polycystic kidney disease *(APKD)*. APKD is an autosomal dominant disease, so anyone who has a K gene has APKD. In this example, the father *(Kk)* has APKD, but the mother *(kk)* does not. How can polymorphism and linkage be used to counsel these parents about the likelihood of APKD in their offspring? Assume that an RFLP (an A allele or an a allele) is found at a locus that is 10 cM from K or k so that the RFLP can be used as a genetic marker. The key to this question is to convert the centimorgan value to a percentage (see Table 11-1). There are four possibilities to consider: 1) If the offspring has the A allele, then there is a **90% chance** that he will inherit the K gene and have **APKD.** The 90% figure is determined by subtracting the chance of crossover between loci (10 cM = 10%) from 100% (100% − 10% = 90%). 2) If the offspring has the a allele, then there is only a **10% chance** that she will inherit the K gene and have **APKD.** The 10% figure is determined by knowing that the distance between the two loci is 10 cM (10 cm = 10%). The chance of crossover between the loci is 10%. 3) If the offspring has the A allele, then there is only a **10% chance** that he will inherit the k gene and be **normal.** The 10% figure is determined by knowing that the distance between the two loci is 10 cM (10 cm = 10%). The chance of crossover between the loci is 10%. 4) If the offspring has the a allele, then there is a **90% chance** that she will inherit the k gene and therefore be **normal.** The 90% figure is determined by subtracting the chance of crossover between loci (10 cM = 10%) from 100% (100% − 10% = 90%). In this way, polymorphism and linkage can be used to counsel these parents about the chances that their offspring will have APKD.

2. Example 2

  a. Question: What is the genotype frequency of heterozygous carriers for sickle cell anemia among black Americans if the S and s allele frequencies are p = 0.96 and q = 0.04, respectively?

  b. Solution: Heterozygous carriers have a genotype of Ss. The genotype frequency of Ss = 2pq. Therefore, $2 \times 0.96 \times 0.04 = 0.0768$, or 7.68%. Dividing $100/7.68 = 13.02$. Therefore, the frequency of heterozygous carriers for sickle cell anemia is 7.68%, or 1 of 13 black Americans.

3. Example 3

  a. Question: What is the genotype frequency of sickle cell anemia in the black American population if the S and s allele frequencies are p = 0.96 and q = 0.04, respectively?

  b. Solution: Because sickle cell anemia is an autosomal recessive disease, black Americans who are affected by this disease have a genotype of ss. The genotype frequency of ss = q^2. Therefore, $0.04^2 = 0.0016$, or 0.16%. Dividing $100/0.16 = 625$. Therefore, the frequency of sickle cell anemia is 0.16%, or 1 of 625 black Americans.

4. Example 4

  a. Question: If the frequency of sickle cell anemia in the black American population is 1 of 625, what is the allele frequency (q) of the s allele?

  b. Solution: If the genotype frequency of the ss genotype (i.e., an individual who has sickle cell anemia) is 1 of 625, then $1/625 = 0.0016$. Because the genotype frequency of the ss genotype = q^2, then $q^2 = 0.0016$. Taking the square root, q = 0.04. Therefore, the allele frequency (q) of the s allele is 0.04.

D. According to the **mutation-selection equilibrium,** gene frequencies in a population are maintained in equilibrium by mutation that replaces abnormal genes that are selectively lost by death **(genetically lethal disease)** or reproductive failure.

1. Autosomal dominant disease

  a. If every carrier of an abnormal gene **dies or cannot reproduce,** then every new case arises from a **new mutation.** Therefore, if the number of people with the disease is **D** and the number of people in the population studied is **N,** then the **disease frequency = D/N** and the **mutation frequency = D/2N.**

  b. Example

   (1) Question: In a study of achondroplasia, 7 new cases were documented among 250,000 births. What are the disease frequency and the mutation frequency?

   (2) Solution: The disease frequency = D/N = $7/250{,}000 = 0.00003$, or 3.0×10^{-5}, or 0.003%. Dividing $100/0.003 = 33{,}333$. Therefore, the disease frequency is 0.00003, or 3.0×10^{-5}, or 0.003%, or 1 of 33,333 people. The mutation frequency = D/2N = $7/2(250{,}000) = 0.000014$, or 1.4×10^{-5}, or 0.0014%. Dividing $100/0.0014 = 71{,}428$. Therefore, the mutation frequency is 0.000014 or 1.4×10^{-5}, or 0.0014%, or 1 of 71,428 people.

2. X-linked recessive disease (genetically lethal in males)

  a. If every carrier of the abnormal gene **dies or cannot reproduce,** then every new case must arise from a **new mutation.** Therefore, if the number of people with the disease is **D** and the number of people in the population studied is **N,** then the **disease frequency = D/N** and the **mutation frequency = D/3N.** (The mutation frequency is D/3N because in a population of equal numbers of males and females, only one-third of the X chromosomes occur in the male and two-thirds occur in the female.)

  b. Example: In a study of fragile X syndrome, 15 new cases in boys were documented among 250,000 births.

   (1) Question: What are the disease frequency and the mutation frequency?

(2) **Solution:** The disease frequency = D/N = 15/250,000 = 0.00006, or 6.0×10^{-5}, or 0.006%. Dividing 100/0.006 = 16,666. Therefore, the disease frequency is 0.00006, or 6.0×10^{-5}, or 0.006%, or 1 of 16,666 people. The mutation frequency = D/3N = 15/3(250,000) = 0.00002, or 2.0×10^{-5}, or 0.002%. Dividing 100/0.002 = 50,000. Therefore, the mutation frequency is 0.00002, or 2.0×10^{-5}, or 0.002%, or 1 of 50,000 people.

E. Genetic drift and the founder effect

1. **Genetic drift** is the random fluctuation of allele frequency in a small population because the pool of genes passed from generation to generation is small.

2. **Founder effect** is a type of genetic drift that occurs in populations that descend from a small number of founding individuals. An allele may occur at a high frequency in the population because it was present in a high frequency among the founders. A well-documented instance is the **Afrikaner population in South Africa,** which descended from a few hundred people who migrated from the Netherlands. The Afrikaner population has a high frequency of Huntington's disease, porphyria variegata, and lipoid proteinosis.

12

Inherited Diseases

I. AUTOSOMAL DOMINANT INHERITANCE

A. Introduction. Diseases that have **autosomal dominant** inheritance affect individuals who have only one defective copy of the gene (from either parent).

B. Example: Huntington's disease (HD) [Figure 12-1]

    1. The characteristic dysfunction is the **cell death of cholinergic neurons and β-aminobutyric acid (GABA) -ergic neurons** within the **caudate nucleus** (corpus striatum). This cell death causes **choreic (dance-like) movements, mood disturbances, and progressive loss of mental activity.** No treatment is available.

    2. The *HD* gene is located on the **short (p) arm of chromosome 4 (4p).**

    3. The *HD* gene encodes for an unknown protein.

    4. The mechanism that causes neuronal cell death in Huntington's disease may involve a **hyperactive N-methyl-d-aspartate (NMDA) receptor.**

        a. Because glutamate is the principal excitatory transmitter in the brain, most neurons have glutamate receptors. One of these receptors is called the **NMDA receptor** because it is selectively activated by the glutamate agonist NMDA.

        b. In normal synaptic transmission, glutamate levels increase transiently within the synaptic cleft. However, neuronal cell death **(glutamate toxicity)** occurs as a result of excessive and diffuse release of glutamate.

        c. Glutamate toxicity is caused by **excessive influx of calcium into the neurons.** This influx is caused by the sustained action of glutamate on the NMDA receptor.

        d. The mutation of the *HD* gene on 4p causes **hyperactivity of the NMDA receptor.** This hyperactivity causes excessive influx of calcium into the neurons of the caudate nucleus, and cell death occurs as a result.

II. AUTOSOMAL RECESSIVE INHERITANCE

A. Introduction. Diseases that have **autosomal recessive** inheritance affect only individuals who have two defective copies of the gene (one from each parent).

B. Example: cystic fibrosis (CF) [Figure 12-2]

    1. The characteristic dysfunction is the **production of abnormally thick mucus** by the epithelial cells that line the respiratory and gastrointestinal tracts. This thick mucus **obstructs the pulmonary airways** and **causes recurrent bacterial respiratory infections.**

    2. The *CF* gene is located on the **long (q) arm of chromosome 7 (7q)** between bands q21 and q31.

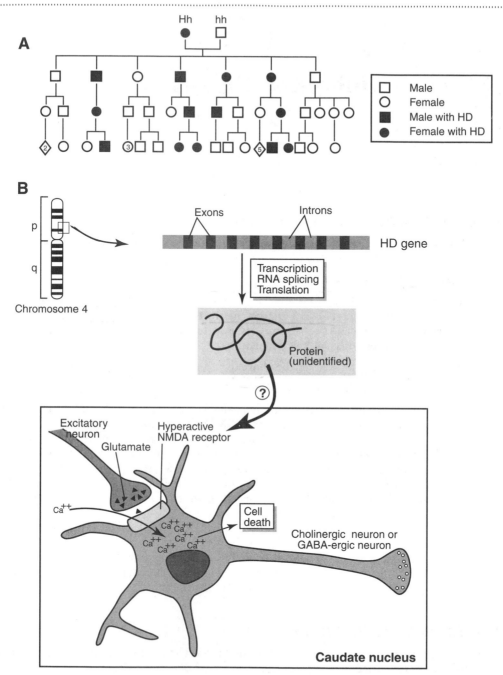

Figure 12-1. (A) Pedigree of Huntington's disease, an example of autosomal dominant inheritance. Heterozygotes (*Hh*) are affected by Huntington's disease. Homozygous recessives (*hh*) are not affected. (Reprinted with permission from Friedman LM: *Genetics*. Malvern, PA, Harwal, 1992, p 46.) (B) Location of the *HD* gene on chromosome 4 (4p). The *HD* gene has not been cloned, and its protein has not been identified. However, the protein may produce a hyperactive N-methyl-d-aspartate (NMDA) receptor that causes excessive influx of calcium into the neurons of the caudate nucleus, causing cell death. *RNA* = ribonucleic acid; *GABA* = β-aminobutyric acid.

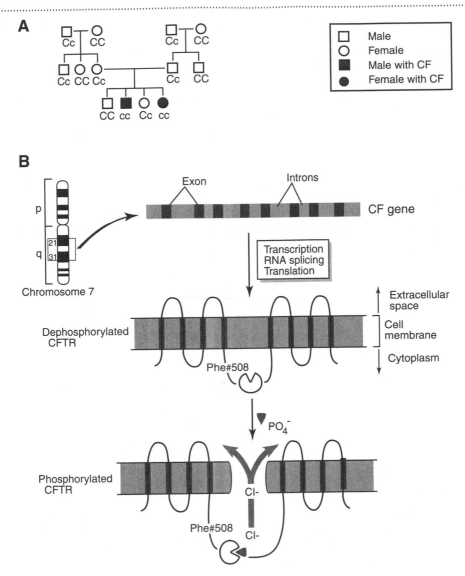

Figure 12-2. (A) Pedigree of cystic fibrosis, an example of autosomal recessive inheritance. Heterozygotes (*Cc*) are not affected, but homozygous recessives (*cc*) are. (B) Location of the CF gene on chromosome 7 (7q). The CF gene has 24 exons that are separated by numerous introns. The CF gene codes for a 1480–amino acid protein called cystic fibrosis transporter (CFTR). CFTR is a Cl⁻ channel that is regulated by phosphorylation. When CFTR is dephosphorylated, the Cl⁻ channel is closed. When CFTR is phosphorylated, the Cl⁻ channel is open. Mutation often occurs at phenylalanine position 508 (*Phe 508*). RNA = ribonucleic acid.

3. The *CF* gene encodes for a protein called cystic fibrosis transporter **(CFTR)**. This protein functions as a **Cl⁻ ion channel.**

4. A mutation in the *CF* gene destroys the Cl⁻ transport function of CFTR.

5. In North America, 70% of cases of cystic fibrosis are caused by a **three-base deletion** that codes for the amino acid **phenylalanine at position 508.** Because of this deletion, phenylalanine is absent from CFTR.

6. CFTR has several membrane-spanning regions and a central region that binds PO_4^{--}.
   a. In dephosphorylated CFTR, the Cl⁻ channel is closed.
   b. In phosphorylated CFTR, the Cl⁻ channel is open.

III. X-LINKED RECESSIVE INHERITANCE

A. Introduction. Diseases that have X-linked recessive inheritance usually occur only in males because males have only one X chromosome (i.e., they are **hemizygous** for X-linked genes). Heterozygous females are clinically normal, but may have subtle clinical features (e.g., intermediate enzyme levels). These diseases occur in females when one of the two X chromosomes is inactivated during the **late blastocyst stage** to form a **Barr body.** This process is called **dosage compensation.** Inactivation of either the maternally or paternally derived X chromosome is a **random and permanent event.** Dosage compensation involves **methylation of cytosine nucleotides.** If the X chromosome that contains the normal gene is inactivated, the female has one X chromosome with the abnormal gene and therefore has the disease.

B. Example: Duchenne type muscular dystrophy (DMD) [Figure 12-3]

   1. The characteristic dysfunction is **progressive muscle weakness and wasting. Death occurs as a result of cardiac or respiratory failure,** usually in the late teens or twenties.

   2. Duchenne muscular dystrophy is caused by **X-linked recessive mutations** [i.e., males who have only one defective copy of the *DMD* gene (from the mother) have the disease].

   3. The *DMD* gene is located on the **short (p) arm of chromosome X in band 21 (Xp21).**

   4. The *DMD* gene encodes for a protein called **dystrophin.** This protein **anchors the cytoskeleton (actin) of skeletal muscle cells to the extracellular matrix** with a transmembrane protein (α-dystroglycan and β-dystroglycan) and stabilizes the cell membrane.

   5. A mutation of the *DMD* gene destroys the ability of dystrophin to anchor actin to the extracellular matrix.

IV. MITOCHONDRIAL INHERITANCE

A. Introduction. Diseases that have mitochondrial inheritance are caused by mutations in the **mitochondrial DNA (mtDNA).** They are inherited entirely through **maternal transmission** because sperm mitochondria do not pass into the ovum at fertilization.

B. Example: Leber's hereditary optic neuropathy (Figure 12-4)

   1. The characteristic dysfunction is **progressive optic nerve degeneration** that causes **blindness.**

   2. Approximately 50% of all cases involve the **ND4 gene** located on mtDNA and occur when a missense mutation changes **arginine to histidine.**

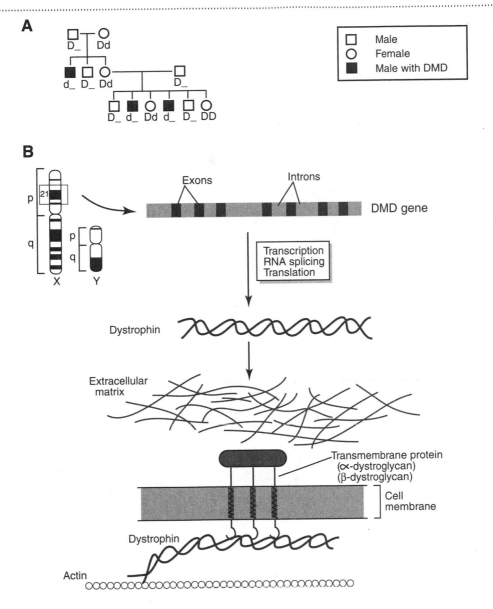

Figure 12-3. (A) Pedigree of Duchenne type muscular dystrophy, an example of X-linked recessive inheritance. Males may be hemizygous for the *DMD* gene (*d_*) because the Y chromosome has no corresponding *DMD* gene. Hemizygous recessive (*d_*) males are affected by Duchenne type muscular dystrophy, but heterozygous (*Dd*) females are not. (B) Location of the *DMD* gene on chromosome X (Xp21). The *DMD* gene consists of exons that are separated by numerous introns. The *DMD* gene codes for a 4000–amino acid protein called dystrophin. Dystrophin anchors actin filaments to the extracellular matrix through a transmembrane protein that consists of α-dystroglycan and β-dystroglycan. *RNA* = ribonucleic acid.

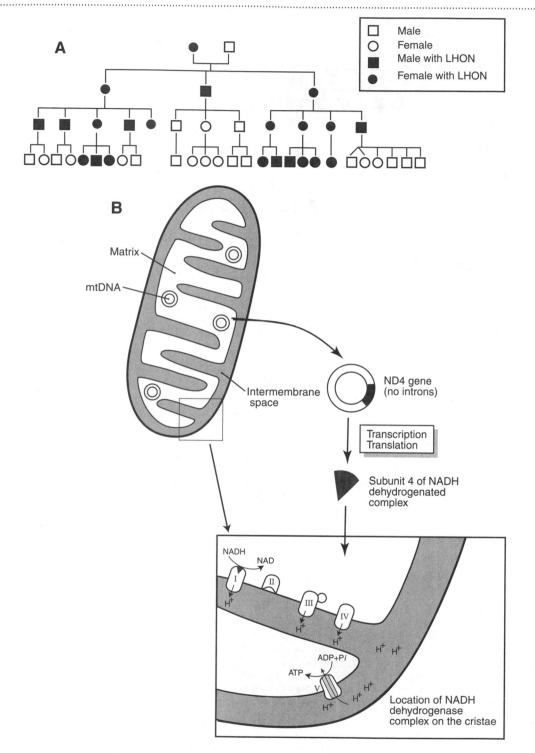

3. The ND4 gene encodes for a protein called **subunit 4 of the NADH dehydrogenase complex** [reduced nicotinamide-adenine dinucleotide (NAD)]. This protein functions in the **electron transport chain** and aids in the **production of adenosine triphosphate (ATP).**

4. A mutation of the ND4 gene decreases ATP production. As a result, the demands of an active neuronal metabolism cannot be met.

V. MULTIFACTORIAL INHERITANCE is discussed in Chapter 13.

VI. TABLE OF INHERITED DISORDERS (Table 12-1)

Figure 12-4.   (A) Pedigree of Leber's hereditary optic neuropathy, an example of mitochondrial inheritance. Leber's hereditary optic neuropathy is inherited maternally. (Reprinted with permission from Friedman LM: *Genetics*. Malvern, PA, Harwal, 1992, p 51.) (B) Location of the ND4 gene on circular mitochondrial deoxyribonucleic acid (*mtDNA*). Like all mitochondrial genes, the ND4 gene contains exons, but no introns. The ND4 gene codes for subunit 4 of the NADH dehydrogenase complex [reduced nicotinamide-adenine dinucleotide (NAD)]. The NADH dehydrogenase complex (I) is shown on the cristae at the start of the respiratory chain (I–IV). The transfer of electrons along the respiratory chain is coupled to adenosine triphosphate (ATP) synthesis. This coupling is caused by the pumping of H^+ into the intermembrane space. The H^+ is subsequently used to drive ATP synthesis. ATP synthesis is catalyzed by ATP synthase (V) as H^+ flows back into the matrix through pores in ATP synthase. II = succinate dehydrogenase; III = ubiquinone-cytochrome c oxidoreductase; IV = cytochrome oxidase; UQ = ubiquinone; ADP = adenosine diphosphate; P_i = inorganic phosphate.

Table 12-1.
Inherited Disorders

Autosomal Dominant Disorders	Autosomal Recessive Disorders	X-linked Disorders	Mitochondrial Disorders	Multifactorial Disorders
α₁-antitrypsin	α-thalassemia	Recessive	Cardiac rhythm disturbance?	Cancer
Achondroplasia	Adrenogenital syndrome	Duchenne type muscular dystrophy	Cardiomyopathy?	Cleft Lip
Actocephalosyndactyly	Albinism	Ectodermal dysplasia	Infantile bilateral striated necrosis	Cleft Palate
Adult polycystic kidney disease	Alkaptonuria	Fabry's disease	Kearns-Sayre syndrome	Clubfoot
Alport's syndrome	Ataxia telangiectasia	Fragile X syndrome	Leber's hereditary optic neuropathy	Congenital heart defect
Bor syndrome	β-thalassemia	Hemophilia A and B		Coronary artery disease
Brachydactyly	Branched chain ketonuria	Hunter's syndrome types A and B		Epilepsy
Cleidocranial dysplasis	Cystic Fibrosis	Ichthyosis		Hemochromatosis
Craniostenosis	Cystinuria	Kennedy's syndrome		Hirschsprung
Crouzon's disease	Dwarfism	Kinky-hair syndrome		Hyperlipoproteinemia types I, IIb, III, IV, V
Diabetes associated with defects in the genes for glucokinase, HNF-1α, and HNF-4α	Erythropoietic porphyria	Lesch-Nyhan syndrome		Hypertension
	Friedreich's Ataxia	Leukocyte G6PD deficiency		Legg-Calve-Perthes disease
	Galactosemia	Testicular feminization		Pyloric stenosis
	Glycogen storage disease	Wiskott-Aldrich syndrome		Rheumatic fever
Ehlers-Danlos syndrome	Hemoglobin C disease	Dominant		Type I diabetes (associated with islet cell antibodies)
Epidermolysis bullosa	Hepatolenticular degeneration	Goltz syndrome		Type II diabetes (associated with insulin resistance and obesity)
Familial Hypercholesterolemia (type IIa)	Histidinemia	Hypophosphatemic rickets		
Goldenhar's syndrome	Homocystinuria	Incontinentia pigmenti		
Heart-hand syndrome	Hypophosphatasia	Orofaciodigital syndrome		
Hereditary spherocytosis	Hypothyroidism			
Huntington's disease	Infantile polycystic kidney disease			
Marfan syndrome	Laurence-Moon syndrome			
Myotonic dystrophy	Lipidosis			
Neurofibromatosis	Mucolipidosis			
Noonan's syndrome	Mucopolysaccharidosis			
Osteogenesis imperfecta	Peroxisomal disorders			
Treacher Collins syndrome	Phenylketonuria			
von Willebrand's disease	Premature senility			
Waardenburg's syndrome	Pyruvate kinase deficiency			
Williams-Beuren syndrome	Retinitis pigmentosa			
	Sickle cell anemia			
	Tyrosinemia			

HNF-hepatocyte nuclear factor.

13

Multifactorial Inherited Diseases

I. DEFINITION. Multifactorial inheritance involves genes that have a small, equal, and additive effect **(genetic component)** as well as an **environmental component.** Both components contribute to the tendency for certain diseases to develop. When only the genetic component of a multifactorial disease is discussed, the term **"polygenic"** is used.

II. EXAMPLE: TYPE I DIABETES (Figure 13-1)

A. The characteristic dysfunction is **destruction of the pancreatic beta cells** that produce insulin. Affected individuals have hyperglycemia, ketoacidosis, and exogenous insulin dependence. Long-term effects include neuropathy, retinopathy that leads to blindness, and nephropathy that leads to kidney failure.

B. Genetic and environmental components

1. Type I diabetes demonstrates **human leukocyte antigen (HLA) association,** specifically with **HLA-DR3** and **HLA-DR4 loci.**

2. These loci are located on the **short (p) arm of chromosome 6 (p6).**

3. The loci code for **cell surface proteins** that are structurally similar to immunoglobulin proteins. They are expressed mainly by B lymphocytes and macrophages.

4. It is hypothesized that genes closely linked to the HLA-DR3 and HLA-DR4 loci may alter the immune response. As a result, affected individuals have an immune response to certain environmental antigens (e.g., a virus). The immune response "spills over" and leads to the destruction of pancreatic beta cells.

5. Markers for this immune destruction of pancreatic beta cells include **autoantibodies to glutamic acid decarboxylase (GAD_{65}), insulin,** and **tyrosine phosphatases IA-2 and IA-2β.** The autoantibodies may destroy the pancreatic beta cells, or they may form after these cells are destroyed.

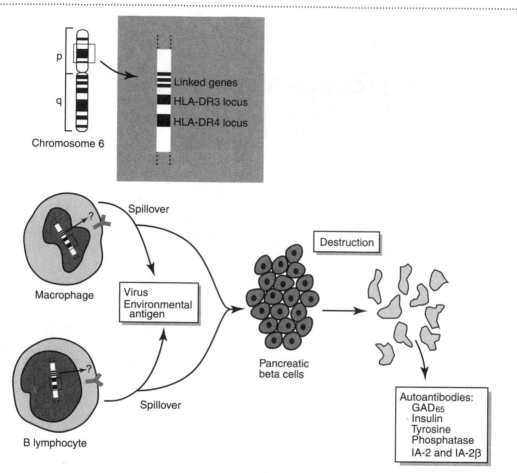

Figure 13-1. Hypothetical model of multifactorial inheritance of type I diabetes. The short (p) arm of chromosome 6 contains the human leukocyte antigen (HLA) complex. The HLA-DR3 and HLA-DR4 loci probably code for cell-surface proteins that structurally resemble immunoglobulins. Genes that are closely linked to these loci may alter the immune response. The nature and role of these linked genes are not known. In response to an environmental antigen, the immune response spills over, and pancreatic beta cells are destroyed. Patients with type I diabetes have serum autoantibodies to glutamic acid decarboxylase (GAD_{65}), insulin, and tyrosine phosphatases IA-2 and IA-2β.

14

Proto-oncogenes, Oncogenes, and Anti-oncogenes

I. DEFINITIONS

A. A **proto-oncogene** is a normal gene that encodes a protein that **stimulates** the cell cycle.

B. An **oncogene** is a mutated proto-oncogene. It encodes an **oncoprotein** that **disrupts** the normal cell cycle and causes **cancer.**

C. An **anti-oncogene (tumor-suppressor gene)** is a normal gene that encodes a protein that **suppresses** the cell cycle.

II. DESIGNATIONS

A. **Proto-oncogenes** and **oncogenes** have italicized three-letter designations, such as *ras*.

B. An **oncogene** that occurs within a **virus** has the prefix "v." An example is **v-*ras*.**

C. A **proto-oncogene** that occurs within a **cell** has the prefix "c." An example is **c-*ras*.**

D. The **protein** that a proto-oncogene or oncogene encodes has the same three-letter designation as the proto-oncogene or oncogene. However, the term is not italicized, and the first letter is capitalized. An example is **Ras.**

III. CLASSIFICATION OF ONCOGENES.

The cell cycle is regulated at four stages (i.e., growth factor, receptor, signal transducer, nuclear transcription). Oncogenes occur at each stage and are grouped into four classes **(Table 14-1).**

IV. MECHANISM OF ACTION OF THE *ras* PROTO-ONCOGENE (Figure 14-1)

A. The *ras* proto-oncogene encodes a normal G protein that has guanosine triphosphatase (GTPase) activity.

B. The G protein is attached to the cytoplasmic face of the cell membrane by the lipid **farnesyl isoprenoid.**

C. When a hormone binds to its receptor, the G protein is activated.

D. The activated G protein binds guanosine triphosphate (GTP), which stimulates the cell cycle.

E. The activated G protein splits GTP into guanosine diphosphate (GDP) and phosphate and terminates the stimulation of the cell cycle.

Table 14-1.
Classes of Oncogenes

Class	Stage	Protein Encoded by Proto-oncogene	Oncogene	Type of Cancer
1	Growth factor	Platelet-derived growth factor	*sis*	Astrocytoma Osteosarcoma
2	Receptors	Epidermal growth factor receptor	*erb*B1	Squamous cell carcinoma of the lung
			*erb*B2	Breast, ovarian, lung, and stomach cancers
			*erb*B3	Breast cancers
3	Signal transducers	Protein tyrosine kinase	*src*	Rous avian sarcoma
		Protein tyrosine kinase	*abl*	Chronic myeloid leukemia, acute lymphoblastic leukemia
		G protein with guanosine triphosphatase activity	*ras**	Human bladder, lung, colon, and pancreas cancers
4	Nuclear transcription factor	Leucine zipper protein	*fos*	Finkel-Biskes-Jinkins osteosarcoma
		Leucine zipper protein	*un*	Avian sarcoma
		Helix-loop-helix protein	N-*myc*	Neuroblastoma
		Helix-loop-helix protein	*myc*	Burkitt's lymphoma
		Retinoic acid receptor (zinc finger protein)	*pml/rarα*+	Acute promyelocytic leukemia

*The *ras* oncogene is found in approximately 15% of all human cancers, including 25% of lung cancers, 50% of colon cancers, and 90% of pancreatic cancers.
+Retinoic acid and the retinoic acid receptor are normally involved in the differentiation of promyelocytes into mature granulocytes. A translocation of the normal retinoic acid receptor gene (*RARα*) from chromosome 17 to the normal promyelocyte gene (PML) on chromosome 15 produces the *pml/rarα* oncogene. The PML/RARα oncoprotein blocks the differentiation of promyelocytes to mature granulocytes. The result is continual proliferation of promyelocytes (i.e., acute promyelocytic leukemia).

F. If the *ras* proto-oncogene mutates, it forms the *ras* oncogene.

G. The *ras* oncogene encodes an abnormal G protein (Ras oncoprotein) in which glycine changes to valine at position 12.

H. Ras oncoprotein binds GTP, which stimulates the cell cycle. Because the Ras oncoprotein cannot split GTP into GDP and phosphate, stimulation of the cell cycle is never terminated.

V. ANTI-ONCOGENES (TUMOR-SUPRESSOR GENES)

A. Retinoblastoma (RB)(Figure 14-2)

1. The RB anti-oncogene is located on chromosome 13. It encodes for the normal **RB protein** that binds to a gene regulatory protein (GRP). As a result, there is no expression of target genes whose gene products stimulate the cell cycle. Therefore, the cell cycle is suppressed.

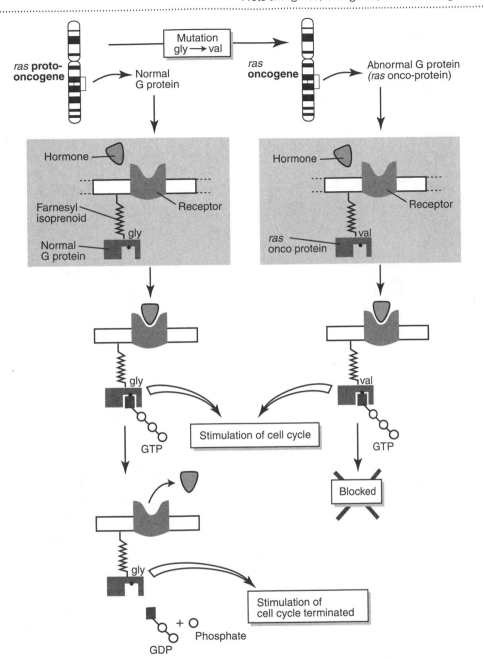

Figure 14-1. Action of the *ras* proto-oncogene. *gly* = glycine; *val* = valine; GTP = guanosine triphosphate; GDP = guanosine diphosphate.

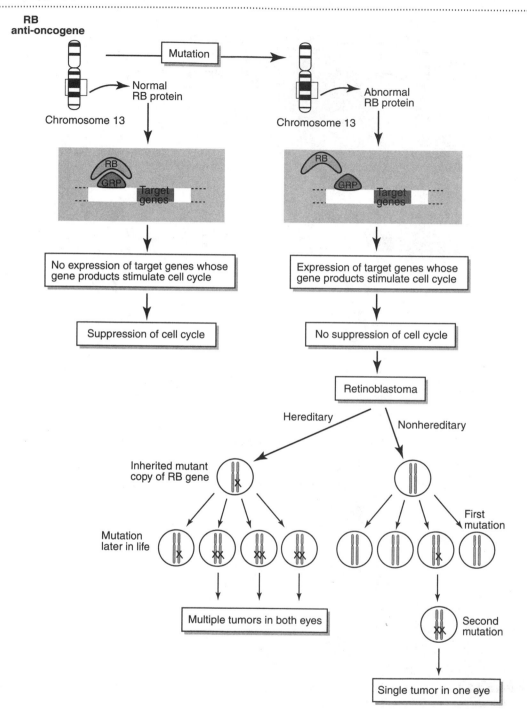

Figure 14-2. Action of the RB anti-oncogene. *GRP* = gene regulatory protein.

2. A mutation of RB encodes an abnormal RB protein that cannot bind to a GRP. As a result, there is expression of target genes whose gene products stimulate the cell cycle. The cell cycle is not suppressed, and a **retinoblastoma** forms.

3. Retinoblastoma occurs in childhood and develops from precursor cells in the immature retina. The **Knudson hypothesis** states that the development of retinoblastoma requires **two separate mutations.** There are two types of retinoblastoma:

    a. Hereditary retinoblastoma

        (1) An affected individual inherits one mutant copy of the *RB* gene.

        (2) Later, a mutation of the second copy of the *RB* gene occurs within **many cells** of the retina. As a result, **multiple tumors** develop in **both eyes.**

    b. Nonhereditary retinoblastoma

        (1) The individual does not inherit a mutant copy of the *RB* gene.

        (2) A mutation of both copies of the *RB* gene occurs within **one cell** of the retina. As a result, a **single tumor develops in one eye.**

4. Although retinoblastoma is rare, the *RB* gene is involved in many types of human cancer.

B. p53 (Figure 14-3)

1. The p53 anti-oncogene is located on chromosome 17. It encodes for the **normal p53 protein (a zinc finger GRP)** that causes the expression of target genes whose gene products suppress the cell cycle at stage **G1** by inhibiting the activity of **Cdk2-cyclin D** and **Cdk2-cyclin E.** As a result, the cell cycle is suppressed.

2. A mutation of p53 encodes an abnormal p53 protein that does not cause the expression of target genes whose gene products suppress the cell cycle. As a result, the cell cycle is not suppressed.

3. Normally, p53 arrests cells that contain damaged deoxyribonucleic acid (DNA) [e.g., by γ-irradiation] in stage G1.

4. The p53 anti-oncogene is the **most common target** for mutation in human cancers.

5. The p53 anti-oncogene is also associated with **Li-Fraumeni syndrome** (an inherited susceptibility to a variety of cancers). Cancer develops in 50% of affected individuals by 30 years of age and in 90% of affected individuals by 70 years of age.

C. Breast Cancer (BRCA 1)

1. The BRCA 1 anti-oncogene is located on chromosome 17. It encodes for **BRCA protein (a zinc finger GRP),** which contains **phosphotyrosine** and suppresses the cell cycle.

2. Between 5% and 10% of women with breast cancer have a mutation of the *BRCA 1* gene. This gene confers a **high lifetime risk** of **breast** and **ovarian cancers.**

D. Other anti-oncogenes are shown in Table 14-2.

VI. MOLECULAR PATHOLOGY OF COLORECTAL CANCER

A. **Most colorectal cancers** develop slowly through a series of histopathologic changes. Each change is associated with a mutation of a specific proto-oncogene or anti-oncogene (Table 14-3).

B. Familial adenomatous polyposis coli (APC)

1. In affected individuals, thousands of polyps develop along the length of the colon early in adult life. If the polyps are not surgically removed, they become malignant. Usually, approximately 12 years elapse from the first detection of polyps to a diagnosis of cancer.

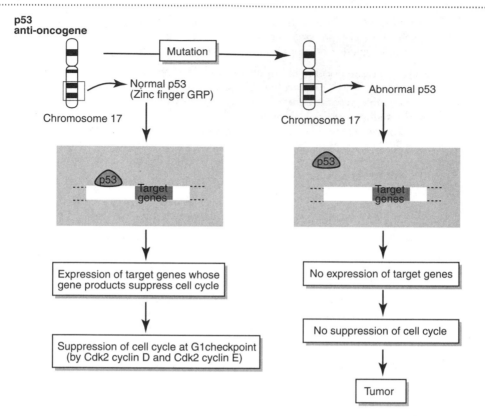

Figure 14-3. Action of the p53 anti-oncogene. *GRP* = gene regulatory protein.

Table 14-2.
Other Anti-oncogenes

Anti-oncogene	Chromosome	Type of Cancer Associated with Mutation
Rb	13	Retinoblastoma, carcinomas of the breast, prostate, bladder, and lung
p53	17	Most human cancers, Li-Fraumeni syndrome
BRCA 1	17	Breast and ovarian cancers
NF-1	17	Schwannoma, neurofibromatosis type 1
WT-1	11	Wilms' tumor
VHL	3	von Hippel-Lindau disease, retinal and cerebellar hemangioblastomas
APC	5	Familial adenomatous polyposis coli, carcinomas of the colon
DCC	18	Carcinomas of the colon and stomach

DCC=deleted in colon carcinoma.

Table 14-3.
Histopathologic Changes Associated with Specific Mutations

Histopathologic Change	Site of Mutation
Normal epithelium to small polyp	APC anti-oncogene
Small polyp to large polyp	*ras* proto-oncogene
Large polyp to carcinoma to metastasis	DCC anti-oncogene p53 anti-oncogene

APC=adonomatous polyposis coli; DCC=deleted in colon carcinoma.

    2. APC involves mutation of the APC anti-oncogene.

    3. APC accounts for 1% of all colorectal cancers.

C. Hereditary nonpolyposis colorectal cancer (HNPCC)

    1. HNPCC **does not** involve mutations of proto-oncogenes or anti-oncogenes.

    2. HNPCC involves a mutation of the **HNPCC gene,** which is the human homologue to the *Escherichia coli* **mutS** and **mutL genes.** These genes code for **DNA repair enzymes** (see Chapter 2).

    3. HNPCC accounts for 15% of colorectal cancers.

15

The Cell Cycle

I. PHASES OF THE CELL CYCLE (Figure 15-1)

A. Gap phase 0 (G_0) is the resting phase of the cell. During this phase, the cell cycle is suspended.

B. Gap phase 1 (G_1)

    1. G_1 is the time between mitosis (M phase) and the synthesis of deoxyribonucleic acid (DNA) [S phase].

    2. Ribonucleic acid (RNA), protein, lipid, and carbohydrate synthesis occurs.

    3. G_1 lasts approximately **5 hours** in a typical mammalian cell with a 16-hour cell cycle.

C. Synthesis (S) phase

    1. DNA and chromosomal protein (eg, histones) synthesis occurs.

    2. It lasts approximately **7 hours** in a typical mammalian cell with a 16-hour cell cycle.

D. Gap phase 2 (G_2)

    1. G_2 is the interval between DNA synthesis (S phase) and mitosis (M phase).

    2. Adenosine triphosphate (ATP) synthesis occurs.

    3. It lasts approximately **3 hours** in a typical mammalian cell with a 16-hour cell cycle.

E. Mitosis (M) phase

    1. Cell division occurs during this phase.

    2. It has six stages:
        a. Prophase
        b. Prometaphase
        c. Metaphase
        d. Anaphase
        e. Telophase
        f. Cytokinesis

    3. It lasts approximately **1 hour** in a typical mammalian cell with a 16-hour cell cycle.

II. CONTROL OF THE CELL CYCLE (see Figure 15-1)

A. **Control proteins.** The two main protein families that control the cell cycle are **cyclin-dependent protein kinases (Cdks)** and **cyclins.** These proteins form **Cdk–cyclin complexes.**

B. **Cdk–cyclin complexes.** The ability of Cdk to phosphorylate target proteins is dependent on the cyclin that forms a complex with it.

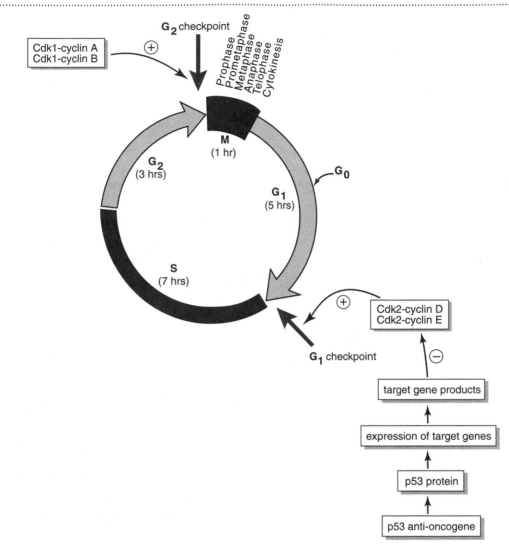

Figure 15-1. The cell cycle with checkpoints. Cdk = cyclin-dependent protein kinase; G_1 = gap phase 1; G_2 = gap phase 2; M = mitosis phase; S = synthesis phase.

   C. Checkpoints are points in the cell cycle where Cdk–cyclin complexes mediate control.

      1. G_1 **checkpoint**
         a. This checkpoint occurs at the $G_1 \rightarrow$ **S phase** transition.
         b. Cdk2–cyclin D and **Cdk2–cyclin E** mediate this transition.
         c. The **p53 anti-oncogene** suppresses the cell cycle at this checkpoint (see Chapter 14)
         d. When this checkpoint operates properly, a cell in the G_1 phase that has **undamaged DNA** enters the S phase through the action of Cdk2–cyclin D and Cdk2–cyclin E. However, a cell in the G_1 phase that has **damaged DNA** (i.e., through mutation, translocation, or rearrangement) is prevented from entering the S phase by the action of the p53 anti-oncogene. Because the damaged DNA is not replicated, the formation of highly transformed, metastatic cells is prevented.

2. G$_2$ checkpoint

   a. This checkpoint occurs at the **G$_2$ → M phase** transition.

   b. **Cdk1–cyclin A** and **Cdk1–cyclin B** mediate this transition.

   c. When this checkpoint operates properly, a cell in the G$_2$ phase that has **undamaged DNA** enters the M phase through the action of Cdk1–cyclin A and Cdk1–cyclin B. However, a cell in the G$_2$ phase that has **damaged DNA** (i.e., through mutation, translocation, or rearrangement) is prevented from entering the M phase. Because cell division does not occur, the formation of highly transformed, metastatic cells is prevented.

D. Inactivation of cyclins

   1. Cyclins are inactivated by **protein degradation** during **anaphase** of the **M phase.**

   2. **Ubiquitin** (a 760–amino acid protein) is covalently attached to the lysine residues of cyclin by the enzyme **ubiquitin ligase.** This process is called **polyubiquitination.**

   3. Polyubiquitinated cyclins are rapidly degraded by proteolytic enzyme complexes **(proteosomes).**

   4. Polyubiquitination occurs widely and marks different types of proteins (e.g., cyclins) for rapid degradation.

III. STAGES OF THE M PHASE (Figure 15-2)

A. Prophase

   1. Chromatin condenses to form well-defined chromosomes.

   2. Each chromosome is duplicated during the S phase and has a specific DNA sequence **(centromere)** that is required for proper segregation.

   3. A **centrosome complex** that acts as the **microtubule organizing center (MTOC)** splits into two halves. The halves move to opposite poles of the cell.

   4. The **mitotic spindle,** which contains microtubules, forms between the centrosomes.

B. Prometaphase

   1. The nuclear envelope is disrupted, giving the microtubules access to the chromosomes.

   2. The nucleolus disappears.

   3. **Kinetochores (protein complexes)** assemble at each centromere on the chromosomes.

   4. Certain microtubules of the mitotic spindle bind to the kinetochores **(kinetochore microtubules).**

   5. Other microtubules of the mitotic spindle are **polar microtubules** and **astral microtubules.**

C. Metaphase

   1. Chromosomes align at the **metaphase plate.**

   2. Cells can be arrested by microtubule inhibitors (e.g., colchicine).

   3. Cells can be isolated for **karyotype analysis.**

Figure 15-2.   Stages of the mitosis (M) phase. (Reprinted with permission from Alberts B, Bray D, Lewis J et al: *Molecular Biology of the Cell,* 3rd ed. New York, Garland Publishing, 1994.)

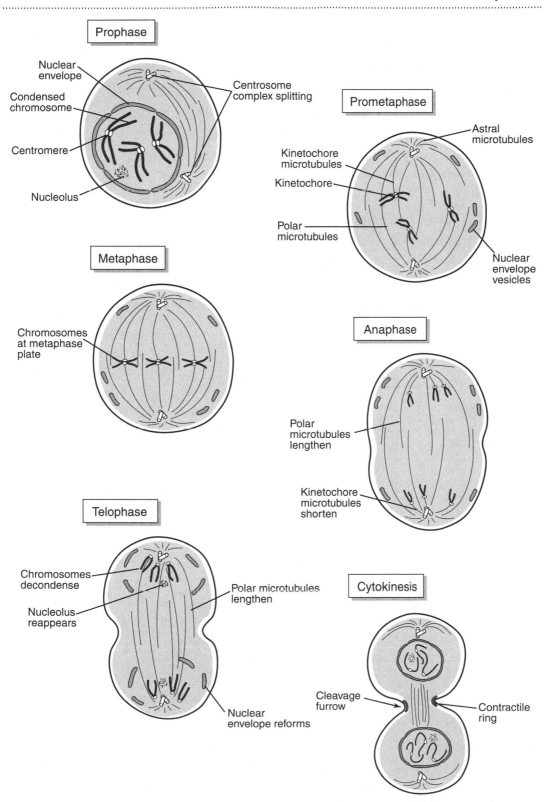

D. Anaphase

    1. The kinetochores separate, and the chromosomes move to opposite poles.

    2. The kinetochore microtubules shorten.

    3. The polar microtubules lengthen.

E. Telophase

    1. Chromosomes decondense to form chromatin.

    2. The nuclear envelope re-forms.

    3. The nucleolus reappears.

    4. The kinetochore microtubules disappear.

    5. The polar microtubules continue to lengthen.

F. Cytokinesis

    1. Cytoplasm divides through the process of **cleavage.**

    2. A **cleavage furrow** forms around the center of the cell.

    3. A **contractile ring** forms at the cleavage furrow. The ring is composed of actin and myosin filaments.

16

Homeotic Genes and Anterior–Posterior Body Pattern Formation

I. INTRODUCTION. In *Drosophila*, bizarre mutations in body pattern occur (e.g., legs sprout from the head in place of antennae). Substitution of one body part for another is called **homeotic mutation.** The genes involved in these mutations are called **homeotic genes.** In *Drosophila*, eight homeotic genes are located in two clusters, called antennapedia (ANT-C) and bithorax (BX-C). These clusters are collectively called the **HOM-complex.** All homeotic genes encode for gene regulatory proteins known as **homeodomain proteins** (see Chapter 7). Homeotic genes contain a 180–base pair sequence **(homeobox)** that encodes a 60–amino acid–long region **(homeodomain).** The homeodomain binds specifically to deoxyribonucleic acid (DNA) segments. Molecular cloning studies show that homeotic genes are highly conserved. Homologues to the HOM-complex in *Drosophila* occur in humans.

II. HUMAN HOMEOTIC GENES

    A. Clustered homeotic genes (Hox-complex) [**Figure 16-1** and **Table 16-1**]. Thirty-nine clustered homeotic genes have been identified in humans. They are organized into four gene clusters **(HoxA, HoxB, HoxC, and HoxD).** These clusters are collectively called the **Hox-complex.** This complex is involved in anterior–posterior body pattern formation in humans. Specifically, it affects the formation of the neural tube, vertebrae, gut tube, genitourinary tract (mesonephric and paramesonephric ducts), limbs, heart tube, and craniofacial area (inner ear and pharyngeal arch 2).

        1. HoxA cluster
            a. This cluster is located on chromosome 7.
            b. It contains 11 genes: HoxA-1, HoxA-2, HoxA-3, HoxA-4, HoxA-5, HoxA-6, HoxA-7, HoxA-9, HoxA-10, HoxA-11, and HoxA-13.

        2. HoxB cluster
            a. This cluster is located on chromosome 17.
            b. It contains 10 genes: HoxB-1, HoxB-2, HoxB-3, HoxB-4, HoxB-5, HoxB-6, HoxB-7, HoxB-8, HoxB-9, and HoxB-13.

        3. HoxC cluster
            a. This cluster is located on chromosome 12.
            b. It contains nine genes: HoxC-4, HoxC-5, HoxC-6, HoxC-8, HoxC-9, HoxC-10, HoxC-11, HoxC-12, and HoxC-13.

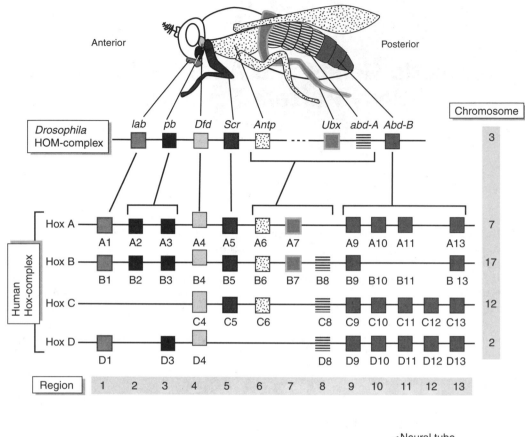

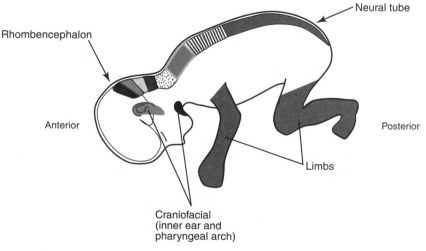

4. HoxD cluster
  a. This cluster is located on chromosome 2.
  b. It contains nine genes: HoxD-1, HoxD-3, HoxD-4, HoxD-8, HoxD-9, HoxD-10, HoxD-11, HoxD-12, and HoxD-13.

B. Nonclustered (divergent, or dispersed) homeotic genes (see Table 16-1) are randomly dispersed throughout the human genome. Because the Hox-complex genes are never expressed anterior to the rhombencephalon, the mesencephalon and prosencephalon derivatives of the human brain involve nonclustered homeotic genes.

Figure 16-1. Relation between the *Drosophila* HOM-complex and the human Hox-complex. Each shaded box represents a homeotic gene on a chromosome. The expression of the various homeotic genes within the body segments of the *Drosophila* and human fetus is shown. A striking feature of the HOM-complex and the Hox-complex is that the order of genes on each chromosome corresponds to the order in which the genes are expressed along the anterior–posterior axis of the human fetus. In the human fetus, *HoxA-2* is the homeotic gene that is expressed most anteriorly (up to the rhombencephalon). No Hox-complex gene is expressed anterior to the rhombencephalon. Examination of the sequence of the Hox-A cluster on chromosome 7 shows that *HoxA-1* should be expressed most anteriorly, but it is not. The homeotic genes are expressed out of sequence (*HoxA-2* is expressed most anteriorly). Abd-A = abdominal-A; Abd-B = abdominal-B; Antp = antennapedia; Dfd = deformed; lab = labial; pb = proboscipedia; Scr = sex combs reduced; Ubx = ultrabithorax. (Adapted with permission from Mark M, Rijli FM, Chambon P: Homeobox genes in embryogenesis and pathogenesis. *Pediatr Res* 42(4):421–429, 1997.)

Table 16-1.

Clinical Features of Clustered and Nonclustered Homeotic Genes in Humans

Homeotic Gene	Associated Clinical Defect
Clustered	
HoxA-1	Inner ear anomalies
HoxA-2	Transformation of pharyngeal arch 2 into pharyngeal arch 1, with duplication of malleus and incus
HoxA-3	Hypoparathyroidism, thymic hypoplasia, thyroid hypoplasia; defective aortic and pulmonic valves, persistent truncus arteriosus, hypertrophy of atria, and thickening of left ventricular wall
HoxA-9	Acute myeloid leukemia
HoxA-10	In males: hypofertility, cryptorchidism, malformation of vas deferens; In females: malformation of uterus
HoxA-13	Hand-foot-genital syndrome (malformation of thumb and great toe, bicarnate uterus, ectopic ureter openings, and hypospadias)
HoxB-2	Facial nerve (CN VII; cranial nerve of pharyngeal arch 2) motor nucleus deficiency, resulting in paralysis of facial muscles (similar to Bells palsy and Möbius' syndrome)
HoxD-13	Synpolydactyly (fusion of fingers or toes)
Nonclustered	
Emx-2	Shizencephaly (absence of large portions of brain and formation of cerebrospinal fluid–filled cleft)
Otx-1	Epilepsy associated with cortical dysgenesis
En-1 and En-2	Agenesis of cerebellum and cerebellar foliation
Pax-3	Type I (malposition of eyelid, hearing impairment, differences in iris coloration, growing together of eyebrows, white forelock of hairs and patchy hypopigmentation) and Waardenburg's syndrome, rhabdomyosarcoma (skeletal muscle neoplasm; the most common soft tissue sarcoma of childhood and adolescence)
Pax-6	Aniridia, Peters anomaly (defect in anterior chamber of eye, with attachment of lens and cornea)
Msx-1	Tooth agenesis (absence of second premolars and third molars)
Msx-2	Boston-type craniosynostosis (but not the more common craniosynostotic syndromes, such as Crouzon syndrome and Apert syndrome, which are caused by mutations in the bibroblast growth factor receptor give)
Rieg	Rieger's syndrome (hypodontia, abnormalities of interior chamber of eye and protuberant umbilicus)
Pit-1	Combined pituitary hormone deficiency (dwarfism)
Pou3f4	Deafness, with fixation of stapes
Pbx-1	Pre-B–cell acute lymphoblastic leukemia
Hox11	T-cell acute lymphoblastic leukemia
Shot and Ogi2x	de Lange's syndrome (mental retardation, growing together of the eyebrows, low forehead, depression of the bridge of the nose, and small head with low-set ears)
Gbx and Nkx3.1	Prostatic cancer

17

Mitochondrial Genes

I. INTRODUCTION. Mitochondrial deoxyribonucleic acid (mtDNA) is a circular segment of DNA that is maternally inherited. The mtDNA contains 16,569 base pairs and is located within the **mitochondrial matrix.** Human mtDNA genes **contain only exons.**

II. GENE PRODUCTS THAT ARE ENCODED BY MITOCHONDRIAL DNA (mtDNA) (Figure 17-1)

A. Ribonucleic acid (RNA)

   1. Two ribosomal RNAs (rRNAs).

   2. Twenty-two transfer RNAs (tRNAs), corresponding to each amino acid.

B. Proteins. The 13 proteins that are encoded by mtDNA are not complete enzymes, but **subunits of multimeric enzyme complexes.** These complexes are used in electron transport and adenosine triphosphate (ATP) synthesis. The 13 proteins are encoded by mtDNA and synthesized on **mitochondrial ribosomes.**

   1. Seven subunits of the reduced nicotinamide-adenine dinucleotide (NADH) dehydrogenase complex.

   2. Three subunits of the cytochrome oxidase complex.

   3. Two subunits of the F_0 adenosine triphosphate (ATP) synthase.

   4. One subunit (cytochrome b) of the ubiquinone–cytochrome c oxidoreductase complex.

III. OTHER MITOCHONDRIAL PROTEINS

A. All other mitochondrial proteins (e.g., enzymes of the citric acid cycle, DNA polymerase, RNA polymerase) are **encoded by nuclear DNA, synthesized on cytoplasmic ribosomes,** and **imported into the mitochondria.**

B. Chaperone proteins, such as **cytoplasmic hsp70, matrix hsp70,** and **hsp60,** aid in the importation of proteins into the mitochondria. Chaperone proteins maintain each protein in an **unfolded state** during importation.

C. The unfolded proteins enter the mitochondria through an **import channel (ISP42).**

IV. MITOCHONDRIAL DISEASES. Mitochondrial diseases show a wide degree of severity. This variability is caused, in part, by the mixture of normal and mutant mtDNA that is present in a particular cell type **(heteroplasmy).** When a cell undergoes mitosis, the

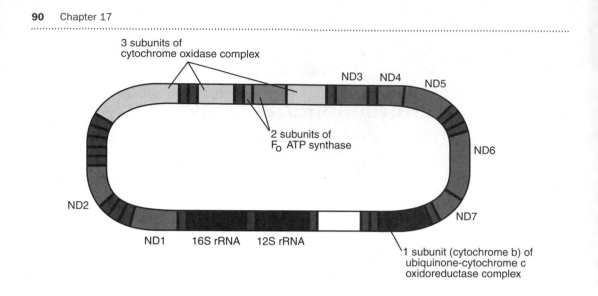

Figure 17-1. Location of mitochondrial deoxyribonucleic acid (mtDNA) genes and their gene products. The shaded areas show the genes for 22 transfer ribonucleic acids (tRNAs). ATP = adenosine triphosphate; F_0 = component of ATP synthase that is sensitive to oligomycin; ND1–7 = genes for the seven subunits of the reduced nicotinamide-adenine dinucleotide (NADH) dehydrogenase complex; rRNA = ribosomal RNA; tRNA = transfer RNA.

mitochondria segregate randomly in the daughter cells. Therefore, one daughter cell may receive mostly mutated mtDNA and the other daughter cell may receive mostly normal mtDNA. In addition, mitochondrial diseases affect tissues that have a **high requirement for ATP, like nerve and skeletal muscle.** Mitochondrial diseases include the following:

A. Leber's hereditary optic neuropathy (see Chapter 11)

B. Kearns-Sayre syndrome, which is characterized by ophthalmoplegia (degeneration of the motor nerves of the eye), pigmentary degeneration of the retina, complete heart block, short stature, and cerebellar ataxia.

C. Myoclonic epilepsy with ragged red fibers syndrome is characterized by myoclonus (muscle twitching), seizures, cerebellar ataxia, and mitochondrial myopathy. The most consistent pathological finding in mitochondrial myopathy is abnormal mitochondria within skeletal muscle that impart an irregular shape and blotchy red appearance to the muscle cells, hence the term **ragged red fibers.**

18
Molecular Immunology

I. THE CLONAL SELECTION THEORY is the most widely accepted theory to explain the immune system. The theory has four major points.

A. B cells and T cells of all antigen specificities develop **before exposure to antigen** occurs.

B. Each B cell carries on its surface an **immunoglobulin** for a **single antigen.** Each T cell carries on its surface a **T-cell receptor** (TcR) for a **single antigen.**

C. B cells and T cells are stimulated by antigens to produce progeny cells that have identical antigen specificity **(clones).**

D. B cells and T cells that react with "self" antigens are eliminated, perhaps through **apoptosis,** or are somehow inactivated so that an autoimmune reaction does not occur.

II. THE B LYMPHOCYTE (B CELL)

A. **Immunoglobulin structure and gene rearrangement (Figure 18-1).** An immunoglobulin has four protein subunits that consist of **two heavy chains** and **two light chains.** The chains are arranged in a Y pattern.

1. Heavy chains
   a. The heavy-chain gene segments are located on chromosome 14.
   b. The heavy-chain gene segments include **200 variable segments** (V_H), **50 diversity segments** (D_H), **6 joining segments** (J_H), and **5 constant segments** (C_H).
   c. The five C_H segments are μ **(mu; M),** δ **(delta; D),** γ **(gamma; G),** ϵ **(epsilon; E),** and α **(alpha; A).** These five segments define the five immunoglobulin (Ig) classes: IgM, IgD, IgG, IgE, and IgD.
   d. V_H, D_H, J_H, and C_H gene segments undergo gene rearrangement to contribute to immunoglobulin diversity.

2. Light chains
   a. The κ **(kappa) chain**
      (1) The κ chain gene segments are located on chromosome 2.
      (2) The κ chain gene segments include approximately **200 variable segments** (V_κ), **5 joining segments** (J_κ), and **1 constant segment** (C_κ).
      (3) The V_κ, J_κ, and C_κ **gene segments** undergo gene rearrangement to contribute to immunoglobulin diversity.
   b. The λ **(lambda) chain**
      (1) The λ chain gene segments are located on chromosome 22.
      (2) The λ chain gene segments include **approximately 100 variable segments** (V_λ), **6 joining segments** (J_l), and **6 constant segments** (C_λ).
      (3) The V_λ, J_λ, and C_λ gene segments undergo gene rearrangement to contribute to immunoglobulin diversity.

A

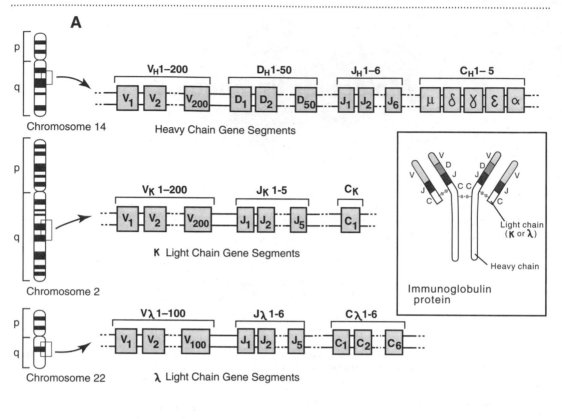

Chromosome 14 — Heavy Chain Gene Segments

K Light Chain Gene Segments

Chromosome 2

λ Light Chain Gene Segments

Immunoglobulin protein

B

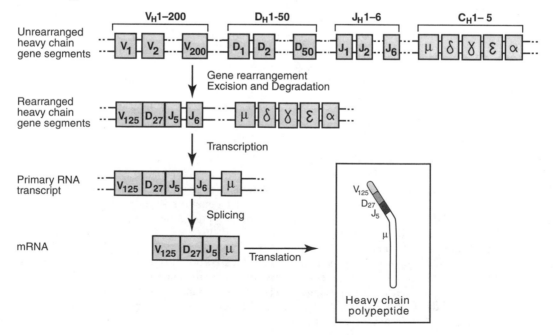

Unrearranged heavy chain gene segments

Gene rearrangement Excision and Degradation

Rearranged heavy chain gene segments

Transcription

Primary RNA transcript

Splicing

mRNA

Translation

Heavy chain polypeptide

3. Gene rearrangement and antibody diversity. For years, the fundamental mystery of the immune system was **antibody diversity:** How could cells of the immune system synthesize a million different immunoglobulins, one for each of the million different antigens? If each immunoglobulin were encoded by its own gene, then the human genome would consist almost exclusively of genes that are dedicated to immunoglobulin synthesis. This is not the case. One of the answers to this fundamental mystery lies in the process of **gene rearrangement,** whereby **V, D, J,** and **C gene segments** of the **heavy** and **light chains** are **randomly rearranged** in a million combinations that code for a million different immunoglobulins. Other processes that play a role in antibody diversity are the presence of **multiple V gene segments in the germ line; random assortment of heavy and light chains; junctional diversity,** whereby DNA deletions occur during gene rearrangement that lead to amino acid changes; **insertional diversity,** whereby a short sequence of nucleotides is inserted during gene rearrangement, leading to amino acid changes; and **somatic cell mutations,** whereby V gene segments mutate during the life of a B cell.

B. **Development of the B cell before exposure to antigen**

1. In early fetal development, B-cell differentiation occurs in the **fetal liver.** In later fetal development and throughout adult life, B-cell differentiation occurs in the bone marrow. In humans, the **bone marrow is the primary site of B-cell differentiation.**

2. **Stem cells** that originate in the bone marrow differentiate into **pro-B cells.**

3. **Pro-B cells** begin D_H to J_H heavy-chain gene rearrangement.

4. **Pre-B cells** begin V_H, D_H, and J_H heavy-chain gene rearrangement.

5. **Immature B cells** (IgM^+) begin light-chain gene rearrangement and express **antigen-specific IgM** (i.e., recognize only one antigen) on their surface.

6. **Mature (virgin) B cells** ($IgM^+ IgD^+$) express antigen-specific IgM and IgD on their surface.

7. Mature B cells migrate to the spleen, lymph nodes, and gut-associated lymphoid tissue (e.g., tonsils, Peyer's patches) and await antigen exposure.

C. **Development of the B cell after exposure to antigen**

1. Early in the immune response, mature B cells bind antigen with IgM and IgD. As a result of this binding, two transmembrane proteins **(CD79a and CD79b)** that function as signal transducers cause B cells to proliferate and differentiate into **plasma cells that secrete either IgM or IgD.**

2. Later in the immune response, mature B cells internalize the antigen–IgM complex or antigen–IgD complex. The complex then undergoes lysosomal degradation in the **endosomal acid vesicles.**

Figure 18-1. (A) Location of heavy-chain and light-chain gene segments on chromosomes 14, 2, and 22. The heavy-chain and light- chain gene segments are organized into various variable (V), diversity (D), joining (J), and constant (C) gene segments. These segments undergo gene rearrangement, transcription, splicing, and translation to form an immunoglobulin protein. An immunoglobulin protein has either two κ light chains or two λ light chains (never one κ light chain and one λ light chain). (B) Rearrangement and immunoglobulin diversity with heavy-chain gene segments. Unrearranged heavy-chain gene segments that have 200 V_H segments, 50 D_H segments, 6 J_H segments, and 5 C_H segments undergo rearrangement. Certain segments (e.g., V_{125}, D_{27}, and J_5) are joined, and the intervening segments are excised and degraded. The rearranged heavy-chain gene segments undergo transcription to form a primary ribonucleic acid (RNA) transcript. This transcript undergoes splicing to form messenger RNA (mRNA) [V_{125}, D_{27}, J_5, and μ]. The mRNA undergoes translation to form a heavy-chain polypeptide that has a unique amino acid sequence that corresponds to the V_{125}, D_{27}, J_5, and μ gene segment codons. Rearrangement contributes to immunoglobulin diversity. *Black segment* = the portion that binds antigen.

3. Some **antigen peptide fragments** join the **class II major histocompatibility complex (MHC)** and are exposed on the surface of the mature B cell.

4. The degradation peptide–class II MHC is recognized by **CD4⁺ helper T cells** that secrete **interleukin-2 (IL-2).**

5. Under the influence of CD4⁺ helper T cells, mature B cells undergo **isotype switching** and **hypermutation.**

    a. Isotype switching

        (1) Isotype switching is a gene rearrangement process whereby the μ and δ C_H **gene segments** are spliced out and replaced with either γ, ϵ, or α C_H gene segments.

        (2) This switching allows mature B cells to differentiate into plasma cells that secrete **IgG, IgE,** or **IgA,** and appears to be mediated by IL-4 and IFN-α

    b. Hypermutation

        (1) Hypermutation is a process whereby a high rate of mutations occur in the **variable segments** of both the heavy chain (V_H) and the light chain (V_κ or V_λ).

        (2) Hypermutation allows mature B cells to differentiate into plasma cells that secrete IgG, IgE, or IgA that will bind antigen with increasing affinity.

III. THE T LYMPHOCYTE (T CELL)

A. T-cell receptor (TcR) structure and gene rearrangement (Figure 18-2). A TcR has two protein subunits: one α **(alpha) chain** and one β **(beta) chain** or one γ **(gamma) chain** and one δ **(delta) chain.**

1. The α chain

    a. The α chain gene segments include **100 variable segments (V_α), 100 joining segments (J_α),** and **1 constant segment (C_α),** resembling the immunoglobulin light chains.

    b. The V_α, J_α, and C_α gene segments undergo gene rearrangement to contribute to TcR diversity.

2. The β chain

    a. The β chain gene segments include approximately **100 variable segments (V_β), 2 diversity segments (D_β), 15 joining segments (J_β),** and **2 constant segments (C_β),** resembling the immunoglobulin heavy chains.

    b. The V_β, D_β, J_β, and C_β gene segments undergo gene rearrangement to contribute to TcR diversity.

3. The γ chain

    a. The chain gene segments are complex, but they contain **variable segments (V_γ), joining segments (J_γ),** and **constant segments (C_γ),** resembling the immunoglobulin light chains.

Figure 18-2. (A) The α, β, γ, δ and chain gene segments. These gene segments are organized into various variable (V), diversity (D), joining (J), and constant (C) gene segments. These segments undergo rearrangement, transcription, splicing, and translation to form a T-cell receptor (TcR) protein. The TcR protein consists of either an α chain and a β chain ($\alpha\beta$) or a γ chain and a δ chain ($\gamma\delta$). (B) Rearrangement and TcR diversity. Unrearranged β chain gene segments with 100 V_β segments, 2 D_β segments, 15 J_β segments, and 2 C_β segments undergo rearrangement. Certain segments (e.g., V_{49}, D_1, J_9, and C_1) are joined, and intervening gene segments are excised and degraded. The rearranged β chain gene segments undergo transcription to form a primary ribonucleic acid (RNA) transcript. This transcript undergoes splicing to form messenger RNA (mRNA) [V_{49}, D_1, J_9, and C_1]. The mRNA then undergoes translation to form a β chain polypeptide that has a unique amino acid sequence that corresponds to the V_{49}, D_1, J_9, and C_1 gene segment codons. *Black segment* = the portion that binds antigen.

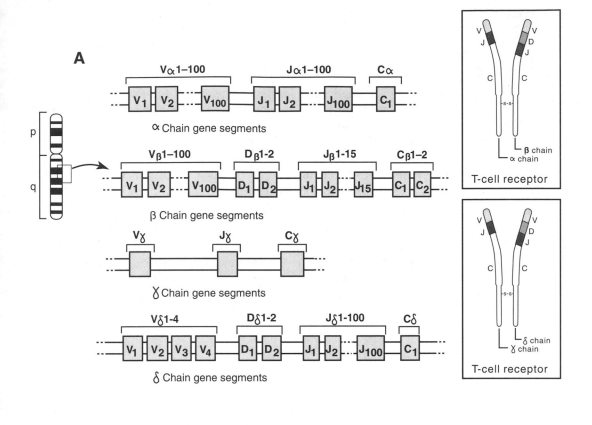

A

$V_\alpha 1-100$ $J_\alpha 1-100$ C_α

V_1 V_2 V_{100} J_1 J_2 J_{100} C_1

α Chain gene segments

$V_\beta 1-100$ $D_\beta 1-2$ $J_\beta 1-15$ $C_\beta 1-2$

V_1 V_2 V_{100} D_1 D_2 J_1 J_2 J_{15} C_1 C_2

β Chain gene segments

V_γ J_γ C_γ

γ Chain gene segments

$V_\delta 1-4$ $D_\delta 1-2$ $J_\delta 1-100$ C_δ

V_1 V_2 V_3 V_4 D_1 D_2 J_1 J_2 J_{100} C_1

δ Chain gene segments

T-cell receptor

T-cell receptor

B

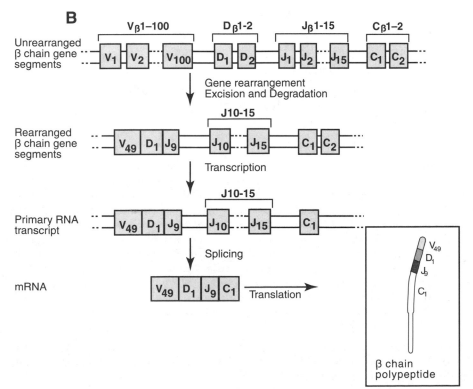

Unrearranged β chain gene segments

$V_\beta 1-100$ $D_\beta 1-2$ $J_\beta 1-15$ $C_\beta 1-2$

V_1 V_2 V_{100} D_1 D_2 J_1 J_2 J_{15} C_1 C_2

Gene rearrangement
Excision and Degradation

Rearranged β chain gene segments

J10-15

V_{49} D_1 J_9 J_{10} J_{15} C_1 C_2

Transcription

Primary RNA transcript

J10-15

V_{49} D_1 J_9 J_{10} J_{15} C_1

Splicing

mRNA

V_{49} D_1 J_9 C_1 Translation

V_{49}
D_1
J_9
C_1

β chain polypeptide

     b. The V_γ, J_γ, and C_γ gene segments undergo gene rearrangement to contribute to TcR diversity.

4. The δ chain
     a. The chain gene segments include approximately **4 variable segments (V_δ), 2 diversity segments (D_δ), 100 joining segments (J_δ),** and **1 constant segment (C_δ)**, resembling the immunoglobulin heavy chains.
     b. The V_δ, D_δ, J_δ, and C_δ gene segments undergo gene rearrangement to contribute to TcR diversity.

5. Gene rearrangement and TcR diversity. The fundamental principles of antibody diversity (see II A 3) also apply to TcR diversity.

B. A **TcR complex** is formed when TcR is expressed on the surface of T cells in association with other transmembrane proteins—most notable among these is **CD3,** which functions as a signal transducer.

C. **Coreceptor proteins.** $\alpha\beta^+$ T cells express two other important transmembrane proteins on their surface. These proteins strengthen the bonds of the TcR–antigen–MHC complex:

     1. **CD4** binds to the invariant portion of **class II MHC protein** and acts as a signal transducer.

     2. **CD8** binds to the invariant portion of **class I MHC protein** and acts as a signal transducer.

D. **Development of the T cell before exposure to antigen**

     1. In early fetal development and until puberty, T-cell differentiation occurs in the **thymus** (derived from **pharyngeal pouch 3**). At puberty, the thymus undergoes **thymic involution,** probably because of increased steroid hormone levels. In humans, the **thymus is the primary site of T-cell differentiation.**

     2. **Stem cells** that originate in the bone marrow migrate into pharyngeal pouch 3.

     3. **Stem cells** differentiate into **pre-T cells** within the **thymic cortex,** where they are protected by the **blood–thymus barrier.**

     4. **Pre-T cells** begin TcR gene rearrangement, and T-cell lineages that express either $\alpha\beta$ TcR or $\gamma\delta$ TcR are established. Much more information is known about the T-cell lineage that expresses the $\alpha\beta$ TcR.

     5. **Immature T cells** express $\alpha\beta$ TcR, CD3, CD4, and CD8 within the thymic cortex.

     6. Immature T cells that express both CD4 and CD8 (**CD4$^+$ CD8$^+$ T cells**) are important intermediate cells because they undergo the following processes:
          a. **Positive selection** is a process whereby CD4$^+$ CD8$^+$ T cells bind with a certain affinity to MHC proteins that are expressed on thymic epitheliocytes. Through this process, the CD4$^+$ CD8$^+$ T cells become **"educated"** to one's own MHC properties. All other CD4$^+$ CD8$^+$ T cells undergo apoptosis. As a result, a mature T cell responds to antigen only when the antigen is presented by an MHC protein that it encountered at this stage in its development **(MHC restriction of T-cell responses).**
          b. **Negative selection** is a process whereby CD4$^+$ CD8$^+$ T cells interact with thymic dendritic cells at the corticomedullary junction of the thymus. CD4$^+$ CD8$^+$ T cells that recognize "self" antigens undergo apoptosis (or are somehow inactivated), thereby leaving CD4$^+$ CD8$^+$ T cells that recognize only foreign antigens.

     7. **Mature T cells** down-regulate CD4 or CD8 to form either $\alpha\beta$ **TcR, CD3$^+$, CD4$^+$, CD8$^-$ T cells** or $\alpha\beta$ **TcR, CD3$^+$, CD4$^-$, CD8$^+$ T cells.** Then they leave the thymic medulla. Mature T cells are never CD4$^+$ CD8$^+$.

8. Mature T cells migrate to the **thymic-dependent zone** of **lymph nodes** and to the **periarterial lymphatic sheath in the spleen,** where they await antigen exposure.

E. Development of the T cell after exposure to antigen

1. **Exogenous antigens** that circulate in the bloodstream are internalized by cells and undergo lysosomal degradation in **endosomal acid vesicles.** Antigen proteins degrade into **antigen peptide fragments** that are presented on the cell surface in conjunction with **class II MHC. CD4⁺ helper T cells** that have the antigen-specific TcR on their surface recognize the antigen peptide fragment.

2. **Endogenous antigens** (viruses or bacteria within a cell) are processed within the **cytoplasm** or **rough endoplasmic reticulum** into **antigen peptide fragments.** These fragments are presented on the cell surface in conjunction with **class I MHC. CD8⁺ killer T cells** that have the antigen-specific TcR on their surface recognize the antigen peptide fragment.

IV. CLINICAL CONSIDERATIONS

A. X-linked infantile (Bruton's) agammaglobulinemia

1. This disorder affects only male infants. It is characterized by recurrent **bacterial** otitis media, septicemia, pneumonia, arthritis, meningitis, and dermatitis. The most common infections are caused by *Haemophilus influenzae* and *Streptococcus pneumoniae*.

2. This disorder occurs at 5 to 6 months of age, when there is an **absence of all classes of immunoglobulins** within the serum.

3. It occurs when pre-B cells cannot differentiate into mature B cells because V_H gene segments do not undergo **gene rearrangement.**

B. Congenital thymic aplasia (DiGeorge syndrome)

1. This disorder is characterized by hypocalcemia and recurrent infections with viruses, bacteria, fungi, and protozoa.

2. It occurs in infants when **pharyngeal pouches 3** and **4** do not develop embryologically. As a result, affected infants have no **thymus** or **parathyroid glands.**

3. These infants have **no T cells.** Many cannot even mount an immunoglobulin response because this response requires CD4⁺ helper T cells.

C. Severe combined immunodeficiency disease (SCID)

1. SCID is a heterogeneous group of disorders. It affects infants and is characterized by a high susceptibility to viral, bacterial, fungal, and protozoan infections.

2. SCID occurs when stem cells do not differentiate embryologically into B cells and T cells.

3. Affected infants have no B cells or T cells. As a result, they seldom survive beyond the first year.

4. **Adenosine deaminase (ADA) deficiency** is a type of SCID in which there is a deficiency of the enzyme ADA. As a result, toxic amounts of adenosine triphosphate (ATP) and deoxyadenosine triphosphate (dATP) accumulate. This accumulation is particularly harmful to lymphoid cells. ADA deficiency is commonly called the **"bubble boy"** disorder. It is the first disorder for which gene therapy was used in humans.

D. Acquired immune deficiency syndrome (AIDS) slowly weakens the immune system through selective destruction of **CD4⁺ helper T cells.**

E. **Monoclonal gammopathies** are a group of **neoplastic** diseases that involve abnormal proliferation of B cells and plasma cells. As a result, excessive amounts of immunoglobulins or immunoglobulin chains are produced.

1. **Multiple myeloma**

a. Multiple myeloma is the most common type of monoclonal gammopathy. It is characterized by high susceptibility to bacterial and viral infections because normal immunoglobulin synthesis is suppressed.

b. It occurs as a result of the **malignant proliferation of plasma cells.**

c. It is associated with **high levels** of **immunoglobulins** (IgM, IgD, IgG, IgE, or IgA), **free κ chains,** or **λ chains (Bence Jones proteins)** in the serum or urine.

2. **Waldenström's macroglobulinemia**

a. This condition is characterized by increased viscosity of the serum, thromboses, disorders of the central nervous system, and bleeding.

b. It is associated with **high levels of IgM.**

19

Receptors and Signal Transduction

I. ION CHANNEL-LINKED RECEPTORS (Figure 19-1) are composed structurally of **multiple subunits** that span the cell membrane. These receptors demonstrate **ion selectivity** (i.e., they permit some ions to pass, but not others). They also have **"gates"** that open briefly in response to stimuli, and then close. Stimuli that open the gates include changes in voltage across the membrane **(voltage-gated ion channels)**, mechanical stress **(mechanical-gated ion channels)**, and neurotransmitters **(transmitter-gated ion channels)**. This chapter discusses transmitter-gated ion channels.

A. Excitatory transmitter-gated ion channels

1. Nicotinic acetylcholine receptor (nAChR)
   a. This receptor has **five subunits.** Each subunit has **two binding sites** for **ACh.**
   b. When nAChR binds **two molecules** of ACh, a conformational change occurs, and the gate opens.
   c. The gate remains open for approximately **1 msec.** While the gate is open, nAChR is nonselectively permeable to all cations (Na^+, K^+, Ca^{++}), but excludes all anions. The **influx of Na^+ ions** (approximately 30,000/msec) is primarily responsible for the **depolarization** of the postsynaptic membrane.
   d. **Nicotine** binds to ACh-binding sites and activates nAChR. For this reason, nicotine is considered an **agonist** and may be responsible for the psychophysical effects of smoking addiction.
   e. **α-Bungarotoxin** and **curare** bind to nAChR and block its action. Therefore, α-bungarotoxin and curare are considered **antagonists.** They cause muscle paralysis when they act at the neuromuscular junction of skeletal muscle.

2. 5-Hydroxytryptamine (5-HT3) serotonin receptor
   a. This receptor is permeable to Na^+ and K^+ ions.
   b. It is widely distributed in the central nervous system (CNS).
   c. It is clinically important because its antagonists have important applications as **antiemetics, anxiolytics,** and **antipsychotics.**

3. Glutamate receptors
   a. N-methyl-D-aspartate (NMDA) receptor
      (1) This receptor is permeable to Na^+, K^+, and Ca^{++} ions.
      (2) Opening the gate requires both **gluta**mate **binding** and **voltage-dependent membrane depolarization** because the NMDA receptor is "plugged" by **extracellular Mg^{++} ions** at resting membrane potential.
      (3) The NMDA receptor is clinically important because its antagonists, such as **phencyclidine (PCP)** and **dizocilpine (MK-801),** may mediate **hallucinogenic behavior.** These antagonists require the NMDA receptor to be opened to gain access to their binding sites. For this reason, they are called **"open-channel blockers."**

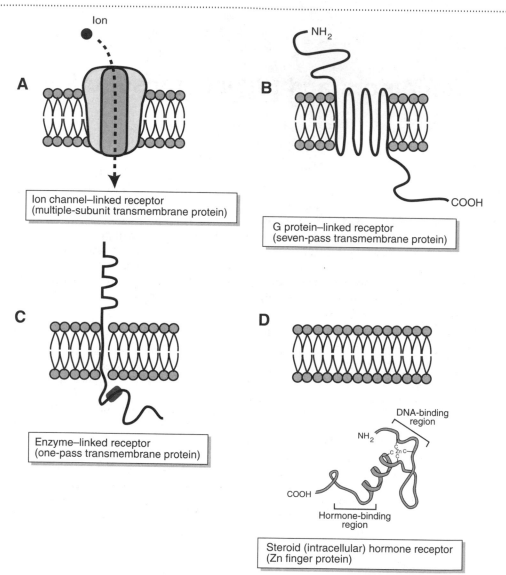

Figure 19-1.   Four classes of receptors.(A) Ion channel–linked receptor (multiple-subunit transmembrane protein). (B) G-protein–linked receptor (seven-pass transmembrane protein). (C) Enzyme-linked receptor (one-pass transmembrane protein).(D) Steroid (intracellular) hormone receptor (zinc finger protein). *DNA* = deoxyribonucleic acid; *C* = cysteine; *Zn* = zinc.

(4) This receptor is clinically important because its hyperactivity causes excessive influx of Ca^{++} ions (**"glutamate toxicity"**). This influx is implicated in many **neurodegenerative disorders.**

(5) This receptor is involved in the **learning process** through **long-term potentiation** in the hippocampus.

B. Inhibitory transmitter-gated ion channels

   1. α-**Aminobutyric acid (GABA$_A$)** receptor

   a. This receptor is permeable to Cl⁻ ions.

b. The influx of Cl⁻ ions is primarily responsible for **hyperpolarizing** the postsynaptic membrane and moving the membrane potential away from the threshold to allow an action potential to occur.

c. It is a major inhibitory receptor within the brain.

d. This receptor is clinically important because **barbiturates** and **benzodiazepines,** such as **diazepam (Valium), chlordiazepoxide (Librium),** and **steroid hormone metabolites** bind to the $GABA_A$ receptor and potentiate GABA binding. As a result, the same amount of GABA causes **increased inhibition** in the presence of these drugs. This increased inhibition may partially mediate the **sedative effects** of these drugs.

e. This receptor is clinically important because its antagonists, such as **picrotoxin, bicuculline,** and **penicillin,** cause **decreased inhibition.** This **decreased inhibition** may mediate the **convulsive** and **seizure activity** of these drugs.

2. Glycine receptor

a. This receptor is permeable to Cl⁻ ions.

b. It is a major inhibitory receptor within the spinal cord.

II. G–PROTEIN–LINKED RECEPTORS (see Figure 19-1) are composed structurally of a **single polypeptide** that spans the cell membrane seven times (seven-pass transmembrane receptors). These receptors are linked to **trimeric guanosine triphosphate (GTP)-binding proteins (G proteins)** that have an α chain, a β chain, and a γ chain. These receptors activate a chain of cellular events through either the **cyclic adenosine monophosphate (cAMP) pathway** or the Ca^{++} **pathway.**

A. cAMP pathway (Figure 19-2A)

1. Increased cAMP levels use stimulatory G (G_s) protein.

a. When the appropriate signal binds to the G_S-protein–linked receptor, **inactive** G_S **protein** [which exists as a trimer with guanosine diphosphate (GDP) bound to the α_S chain] exchanges its GDP for GTP to become **active** G_S **protein.**

b. This change allows the α_S chain to dissociate from the β_S and γ_S chains. The α_S chain stimulates adenylate cyclase to increase cAMP levels.

c. Active G_S protein is short-lived because the α_S chain has **guanosine triphosphatase (GTPase) activity** that quickly hydrolyzes GTP to GDP to form inactive G_S protein.

d. cAMP activates the enzyme **cAMP-dependent protein kinase (protein kinase A),** which catalyzes the **covalent phosphorylation** of serine and threonine within certain intracellular proteins to increase their activity.

e. The enzyme **serine–threonine protein phosphatase** reverses the effects of protein kinase A by dephosphorylating serine and threonine.

f. This process is clinically important because **cholera toxin,** an enzyme that catalyzes the **adenosine diphosphate (ADP) ribosylation** of the α_S chain, blocks α_S chain GTPase activity and permits the effects of active G_S protein to continue indefinitely. Within the intestinal epithelium, this change causes Na⁺ ions and water to move into the gut lumen, resulting in severe **diarrhea.**

2. Decreased cAMP levels use inhibitory G (G_i) protein.

a. When the appropriate signal binds to the G_i-protein–linked receptor, **inactive** G_i **protein** (which exists as a trimer with GDP bound to the α_i chain) exchanges its GDP for GTP to become **active** G_i **protein.**

b. This exchange allows the α_i chain to dissociate from the β_i and γ_i chains and inhibit adenylate cyclase to decrease cAMP levels.

c. This change is clinically important because **pertussis toxin,** an enzyme that catalyzes the **ADP ribosylation of the** α_i **chain,** blocks the dissociation of the α_i chain from the β_i and γ_i chains. As a result, adenylate cyclase is not inhibited.

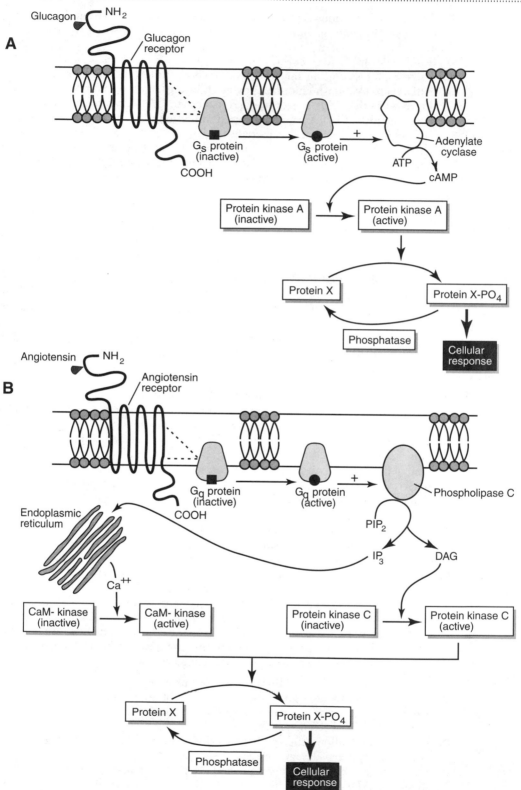

B. Ca^{++} pathway (see Figure 19-2B)

1. When the appropriate signal binds to the G$_q$-protein–linked receptor, **inactive Gq protein** (which exists as a trimer with GDP bound to the γ chain) exchanges its GDP for GTP to become **active G$_q$ protein.**

2. Active G$_q$ protein activates **phospholipase C,** which cleaves **phosphatidyl inositol biphosphate (PIP$_2$)** into **inositol triphosphate (IP$_3$)** and **diacylglycerol (DAG).**

3. IP$_3$ causes the **release of Ca^{++}** from the endoplasmic reticulum. This release activates the enzyme **Ca^{++}/calmodulin-dependent protein kinase (CaM-kinase),** which catalyzes the **covalent phosphorylation** of serine and threonine within certain intracellular proteins to increase their activity.

4. DAG activates the enzyme **protein kinase C,** which catalyzes the covalent phosphorylation of serine and threonine within certain intracellular proteins to increase their activity.

C. Types of G-protein–linked receptors

1. **Muscarinic ACh receptor (mAChR)**
   a. This receptor plays a major role in mediating the actions of ACh in the brain.
   b. **Atropine, N-methylscopolamine,** and **pirenzepine** are antagonists of mAChR.

2. **Adrenergic receptors (ARs)** are grouped into three families, all of which bind the catecholamines **epinephrine** and **norepinephrine.**
   a. **α1 AR** uses the Ca^{++} pathway.
   b. **α2 AR**
      (1) α2 AR uses the cAMP pathway and decreases cAMP levels by inhibiting adenylate cyclase.
      (2) α-Adrenergic receptor antagonists include **phentolamine, phenoxybenzamine, prazosin,** and **yohimbine.**
   c. **β1, β2, and β3 ARs**
      (1) These ARs use the cAMP pathway and increase cAMP levels by stimulating adenylate cyclase.
      (2) β-Adrenergic receptor antagonists include **propranolol, metoprolol, atenolol, pindolol, timolol, nadolol, betaxolol,** and **esmolol.**

3. Dopamine receptors
   a. Dopamine receptors are grouped into two main classes **(D1 and D2),** both of which bind the catecholamine **dopamine.**
   b. D1 receptors use the cAMP pathway and increase cAMP levels by stimulating adenylate cyclase.
   c. D2 receptors also use the cAMP pathway. They decrease cAMP levels by inhibiting adenylate cyclase.
   d. These receptors are clinically important in **Parkinson's disease,** a neurodegenerative disorder that causes **depletion of dopamine** within the **substantia nigra** and **corpus striatum.** These areas play a role in coordinating muscle movements.

4. Purinergic receptors
   a. These receptors are grouped into two main classes **(A-type and P-type).**
   b. A-type receptors bind **adenosine.**

Figure 19-2. Signal transduction of G-protein–linked receptors. (A) Cyclic adenosine monophosphate (cAMP) pathway. (B) Ca^{++} pathway. G$_s$ = stimulatory G protein; *ATP* = adenosine triphosphate; G$_q$ = G protein that activates phospholipase; *IP$_3$* = inositol triphosphate; *PIP$_2$* = phosphatidyl inositol biphosphate; *DAG* = diacylglycerol; *ER* = endoplasmic reticulum; *CaM-kinase* = Ca^{++}/calmodulin-dependent protein kinase.

    c. P-type receptors bind **adenosine triphosphate (ATP).**

    d. Adenosine has important modulatory effects on the CNS. Adenosine is highly permeable to the cell membrane and diffuses into and out of neurons easily. This diffusion establishes a feedback loop through which the metabolic status (high or low ATP activity, which leads to an accumulation of adenosine) of a neuron is communicated to surrounding neurons.

5. Metabotropic glutamate receptors (mGluRs)
    a. There are eight types of mGluRs (**mGluR1** through **mGluR8**).
    b. mGluRs are found throughout the CNS.

6. γ-Aminobutyric acid (GABA$_B$) receptor
    a. This receptor is found throughout the CNS, where it colocalizes with the GABA$_A$ receptor (a transmitter-gated ion channel).
    b. Saclofen is an antagonist of the GABA$_B$ receptor.
    c. Baclofen is an agonist of the GABA$_B$ receptor.

7. Thyrotropin (TSH) receptor. A defect in the TSH receptor gene is implicated in **hyperthyroidism (thyroid adenomas).**

8. Luteinizing hormone (LH) receptor. A defect in the LH receptor gene is implicated in **precocious puberty.**

9. Adrenocorticotropic hormone (ACTH) receptor. A defect in the ACTH receptor gene is implicated in **familial glucocorticoid deficiency.**

10. Glucagon receptor

11. Rhodopsin receptor. A defect in the rhodopsin receptor gene is implicated in **retinitis pigmentosa,** a degenerative disease characterized by the development of night blindness (nyctalopia) as a result of the death of rod photoreceptor cells in the retina.

12. Neuropeptide receptors. There are many peptide receptors, some of which are reviewed here.
    a. Vasopressin receptors
        (1) There are two types (V$_1$ and V$_2$).
        (2) A defect in the V$_2$ vasopressin receptor gene is implicated in **X-linked nephrogenic diabetes insipidus.**
    b. Angiotensin receptor
    c. Bradykinin receptor
    d. Neuropeptide Y receptor
    e. Neurotensin receptor
    f. Opiate receptors
    g. Oxytocin receptor
    h. Vasoactive intestinal polypeptide (VIP) receptor

III. ENZYME-LINKED RECEPTORS (see **Figure 19-1**) are composed structurally of **single** or **multiple polypeptides** that span the cell membrane once (one-pass transmembrane receptors). These receptors are unique in that their cytoplasmic domain has **intrinsic enzyme activity** or **associates directly with an enzyme. Receptor guanylate cyclase** activates a chain of cellular events through **production of cyclic guanosine monophosphate (GMP) [cGMP]. Receptor tyrosine kinase** activates a chain of cellular events through the **autophosphorylation of tyrosine. Tyrosine kinase–associated receptor** activates a chain of cellular events through the **phosphorylation of tyrosine. Receptor tyrosine phosphatase** activates a chain of cellular events through the **dephosphorylation of tyrosine. Receptor serine–threonine kinase** activates a chain of cellular events through the **phosphorylation of serine–threonine.**

A. Production of receptor guanylate cyclase (cGMP)

1. When the appropriate signal binds to receptor guanylate cyclase, its intrinsic enzyme guanylate cyclase activity produces cGMP.

2. cGMP activates **cGMP-dependent protein kinase (protein kinase G),** which catalyzes the **covalent phosphorylation** of serine and threonine within certain intracellular proteins to increase their activity.

B. Autophosphorylation of tyrosine (receptor tyrosine kinase; Figure 19-3)

1. When the appropriate signal binds to receptor tyrosine kinase, its intrinsic tyrosine kinase activity catalyzes the **autophosphorylation** of tyrosine and produces **phosphotyrosine** within the receptor.

2. Many intracellular proteins bind to the phosphotyrosine residues. These proteins share a sequence homology **(SH$_2$ domain)** and are called **SH$_2$-domain proteins.**

3. SH$_2$-domain protein interacts with **son-of-sevenless (Sos) protein.**

4. Sos protein activates **Ras protein** by causing Ras protein to bind GTP. Ras protein is a monomeric G protein that is the gene product of the *ras* **proto-oncogene** (see Chapter 14).

5. The activated Ras protein activates **Raf protein kinase.**

6. The activated Raf protein kinase activates **mitogen-activated protein (MAP) kinase** by the covalent phosphorylation of tyrosine and threonine.

7. The activated MAP kinase leaves the cytoplasm and enters the nucleus, where it phosphorylates gene regulatory proteins. These proteins then cause **gene transcription.**

C. Phosphorylation of tyrosine (tyrosine kinase–associated receptor)

1. When the appropriate signal binds to a tyrosine kinase–associated receptor, the tyrosine kinase catalyzes the **covalent phosphorylation** of tyrosine within certain intracellular proteins to increase the activity of the proteins.

2. The **Src protein** is an important tyrosine kinase that is associated with the receptor. This protein is the gene product of the *src* **proto-oncogene** (see Chapter 14).

D. Dephosphorylation of tyrosine (receptor tyrosine phosphatase). When the appropriate signal binds to a receptor tyrosine phosphatase, its intrinsic tyrosine phosphatase catalyzes the **dephosphorylation** of tyrosine within certain intracellular proteins. As a result, the activity of these proteins increases.

E. Phosphorylation of serine–threonine (receptor serine–threonine kinase). When the appropriate signal binds to a receptor serine–threonine kinase, its intrinsic serine–threonine kinase activity catalyzes the **covalent phosphorylation** of serine and threonine within certain intracellular proteins. As a result, the activity of these proteins increases.

F. Types of enzyme-linked receptors

1. Receptor guanylate cyclase: Atrial natriuretic peptide (ANP) receptor

2. Receptor tyrosine kinase:
   a. Epidermal growth factor (EGF) receptor
   b. Platelet-derived growth factor (PDGF) receptor
   c. Fibroblast growth factor (FGF) receptor
   d. Nerve growth factor (NGF) receptor
   e. Vascular endothelial growth factor (VEGF) receptor
   f. Insulin receptor

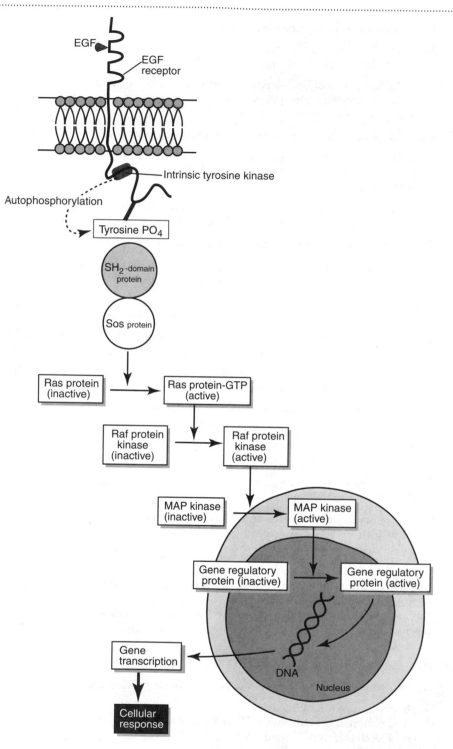

Figure 19-3. Signal transduction of enzyme-linked receptors. *EGF* = epidermal growth factor; *SH₂* = sequence homology protein; *Sos* = son-of-sevenless; *Ras* = rat sarcoma; *MAP* = mitogen-activated protein; *DNA* = deoxyribonucleic acid.

   3. Tyrosine kinase-associated receptor:
   a. Cytokine receptors
   b. Growth hormone receptor
   c. Prolactin hormone receptor
   d. Antigen-specific receptors on B and T lymphocytes
   e. Interleukin-2 (IL-2) receptor

   4. Receptor tyrosine phosphatase: CD45

   5. Receptor serine–threonine kinase: Transforming growth factor β (TGFβ) receptor

IV. STEROID HORMONE (INTRACELLUALR) RECEPTORS (see Figure 19-1) are composed structurally of a polypeptide with a zinc atom that is bound to four cysteine amino acids (**zinc finger protein;** see Chapter 7). These receptors are actually **gene regulatory proteins** that have a **hormone-binding region** as well as a **DNA-binding region** that activates **gene transcription.**

   A. Activation of gene transcription (Figure 19-4)

   1. Inactive steroid hormone receptors are found in the cytoplasm, where they are bound to **heat shock protein 90 (hsp90)** and **immunophilin (hsp56).**

   2. When the appropriate signal (i.e., steroid hormone) **diffuses** across the cell membrane and binds to the hormone-binding region of the steroid hormone receptor, hsp90 and hsp56 are released, and the DNA-binding region is exposed.

   3. The steroid–receptor complex is transported to the **nucleus,** where it binds to DNA and activates the transcription of a small number of specific genes within approximately 30 minutes (**primary response**).

   4. The gene products of the primary response activate other genes to produce a **secondary response.**

   B. Types of steroid hormone (intracellular) receptors

   1. Glucocorticoid receptor

   2. Estrogen receptor

   3. Progesterone receptor

   4. Thyroid hormone receptor

   5. Retinoic acid receptor

   6. Vitamin D_3 receptor

V. RECEPTOR TYPES. Table 19-1 summarizes the types of receptors.

VI. NITRIC OXIDE (NO)

   A. NO is a labile, free radical **gas** with a half-life of about five seconds.

   1. It plays an important role in the **immune function of macrophages.**

   2. It also plays an important role in **blood vessel dilation.**

   3. It serves as a **neurotransmitter** in the central nervous system (CNS) and peripheral nervous system (PNS).

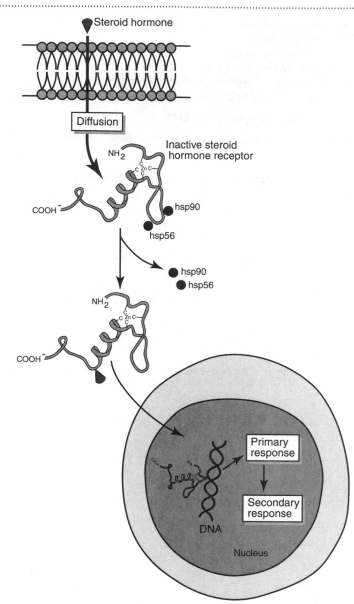

Figure 19-4. Signal transduction of steroid hormone receptors. C = cysteine; Zn = zinc; DNA = deoxyribonucleic acid; hsp = heat shock protein.

B. NO forms through the action of **nitric oxide synthase (NOS),** which catalyzes the reaction that transforms **arginine** into **citrulline and NO.**

C. NO elicits its action by binding to the heme group of a unique cytoplasmic **receptor guanylate cyclase** to produce **cyclic guanosine monophosphate (cGMP).** cGMP activates **protein kinase G,** which catalyzes the covalent phosphorylation of serine and threonine within certain intracellular proteins to increase their activity.

D. NO is the active metabolite that mediates the relaxant effects of many **anti-angina organic nitrates** such as **nitroglycerin** and **nitroprusside;** these organic nitrates are metabolized slowly to produce NO.

Table 19-1.
Types of Receptors

Ion Channel-Linked Receptors	G-Protein-Linked Receptors	Enzyme-Linked Receptors	Steroid Hormone (Intracellular) Receptors
Transmitter-gated ion channel	mAChR	Receptor guanylate cyclase	Glucocorticoid receptor
Excitatory	Adrenergic receptors (α1, α2, β1, β2, β3)	ANP receptor	Estrogen receptor
nAChR			Progesterone receptor
5-HT3 serotonin receptor	Dopamine receptors (D1 and D2)	Receptor tyrosine kinase	Thyroid hormone receptor
Glutamate receptors	Purinergic receptors (A-type and P-type)	EGF receptor	Retinoic acid receptor
NMDA receptor		PDGF receptor	Vitamin D_3 receptor
Kainate receptor	mGluR	FGF receptor	
Quisqualate A receptor		NGF receptor	
AMPA receptor	GABA$_B$ receptor	VEGF receptor	
Inhibitory	TSH receptor	Insulin receptor	
GABA$_A$ receptor	ACTH receptor		
Glycine receptor	LH receptor	Tyrosine kinase-associated receptor	
	Glucagon receptor	Cytokine receptors	
	Rhodopsin receptor	Growth hormone receptor	
		Prolactin receptor	
	Neuropeptide receptors	Antigen-specific receptors	
	Vasopressin receptors	IL-2 receptor	
	Angiotensin receptor		
	Bradykinin receptor	Receptor tyrosine phosphatase (CD45)	
	Neuropeptide Y receptor		
	Neurotensin receptor	Receptor serine–threonine kinase (TGFβ)	
	Opiate receptors		
	Oxytocin receptor		
	VIP receptor		

ACTH = adrenocorticotropic hormone; AMPA = γ-amino-3-hydroxy-5-methylisoxazole propionic acid; ANP = nutriuretic peptide; EGF = epidermal growth factor; FGF = fibroblast growth factor; GABA = aminobutyric acid; 5-ht3 = 5-hydroxytryptamine; IL-2 = interleukin-2; LH = luteinizing hormone; mAChR = muscarinic acetylcholine receptor; mGluR = metabotropic glutamate receptor; nAChR = nicotinic acetylcholine receptor; NGF = nerve growth factor; NMDA = N-methyl-D-aspartate; PDGF = platelet-derived growth factor; TGFβ-transforming growth factor β; TSH = thyrotropin; VEGF = vascular endothelial growth factor; VIP = vasoactive intestinal polypeptide.

E. NO, produced by endothelial cells within the tunica intima of blood vessels, diffuses to the smooth muscles within the tunica media, and causes smooth muscle relaxation; for example, vasodilation.

F. NO is produced by the nerve fibers within the tunica adventia of the **deep cavernous artery of the penis,** as well as nerve fibers around the sinusoids of the **corpora cavernosae of the penis.**

    1. **NO and cGMP** thus play a significant role in penile erection.

    2. Viagra (sildenafil) is an orally active **cGMP phosphodiesterase (Type 5) inhibitor** that promotes high levels of cGMP and vasodilation, and hence, penile erection; Viagra, therefore, has become a popular drug choice for the treatment of penile erectile dysfunction.

VII. RECEPTOR-MEDIATED ENDOCYTOSIS

A. Receptor-mediated endocytosis is a process whereby a certain substance [e.g., **low density lipoprotein (LDL)**] is taken up, or endocytosed by a cell, by means of the action of a specific receptor (e.g., **LDL receptor**). LDL is the principle carrier of serum **cholesterol.**

B. Receptor-mediated endocytosis occurs when:

    1. The LDL receptor binds LDL circulating in the blood to form **clathrin-coated pits** in the cell membrane.

    2. The clathrin-coated pits invaginate to form **clathrin-coated vesicles** that fuse with an **early endosome** or compartment for uncoupling of receptor and ligand **(CURL)** where the LDL receptor and LDL are disassociated from one another. The early endosome fuses with a **late endosome** containing active **lysosomal enzymes.**

    3. The LDL is lysosomally degraded to **cholesterol,** which is released into the cytoplasm.

    4. The cholesterol inhibits the enzyme **3-hydroxy-3-methylglutaryl-CoA (HMG-CoA) reductase,** which catalyzes the committed step in cholesterol biosynthesis and thereby suppresses **de novo** cholesterol biosynthesis.

    5. The process contributes to keeping serum cholesterol levels in the normal range.

C. Receptor-mediated endocytosis is clinically relevant in a condition called **familial hypercholesterolemia (FH).**

    1. FH is a genetic disease involving mutations in the LDL receptor protein, which causes elevated levels of serum cholesterol and increased incidence of heart attack early in life.

    2. There are two types of FH-associated LDL receptor protein mutations:
        a. The LDL receptor fails to bind LDL
        b. The LDL receptor binds LDL, but fails to undergo endocytosis.

    3. In FH, HMG-CoA reductase activity and de novo cholesterol biosynthesis are unchecked.